An Outline of
Rheumatology

Peter Hickling BSc MRCP

Consultant Rheumatologist, Plymouth Health District
Formerly Senior Registrar, Rheumatism Research Unit,
University of Leeds and St James's University Hospital, Leeds

and
John R. Golding DM FRCP

Formerly Consultant Rheumatologist, St James's University
Hospital, Leeds; Clinical Senior Lecturer, University of Leeds

With a Foreword by
Verna Wright MD FRCP
Professor of Rheumatology, University of Leeds

WRIGHT
1984   Bristol

Published by
John Wright & Sons Ltd,
823–825 Bath Road,
Bristol BS4 5NU, England

*British Library Cataloguing in
Publication Data*

Hickling, P.
   An outline of rheumatology.
   1. Rheumatism
   I. Title   II. Golding, J. R.
   616.7'23   RC927

ISBN 0 7236 0769 9

Library of Congress
Catalog Card Number 84–50683

Typeset by Activity Limited,
Salisbury, Wiltshire

Printed in Great Britain by
John Wright & Sons
(Printing) Ltd at
The Stonebridge Press,
Bristol BS4 5NU

An Outline of Rheumatology

Preface

The subject of rheumatology covers a vast number of diseases. It includes some conditions that affect virtually every one of us at some time in our lives. In terms of patient referrals to practitioners, it forms one of the largest disease groups encountered in general medicine. It is thus very important that medical students are exposed to rheumatology at some stage during the course of their training. The medical school curriculum, however, is becoming increasingly crowded as the various subspecialties compete for students' time. Teaching in the subspecialties tends therefore to be very concentrated, and to give a broad overview of the subject in a short time is extremely difficult. This book is intended to overcome that difficulty. Its scope is broad, all the major disease states encountered in rheumatology are discussed. In accordance with its title, however, the authors have attempted to keep the book as clinically relevant as possible, and outline the major facets of each disease rather than dwell on minutiae which the student can hopefully glean from larger tomes. It is intended that the book be read in parallel with a rheumatology teaching programme orientated towards outpatient and bedside teaching, and not read in the sterile atmosphere of the tutorial room or lecture theatre.

Although basically aimed at medical students, it is hoped that this book will be of interest to postgraduate students studying for higher diplomas such as the MRCP and the MRCGP. Members of the nursing profession may also care to dip into it from time to time, to help them further understand the problems of patients with rheumatic diseases under their care.

P.H.
J.R.G.

Acknowledgements

We wish to acknowledge the help of the following people, without whom production of this book would not have been possible. Mrs E.A. Langdon, Mrs C. Shaw, Mrs J. Hodson and Mrs B. Guest for unstinting, accurate and patient secretarial help. Mr B. Emison (Medical Illustration Department, St James's University Hospital, Leeds) and Mr T. Macausland (Medical Illustration Department, Derriford Hospital, Plymouth) for their technical advice and help with illustrations.

Contents

Foreword

By **Verna Wright** MD FRCP
Professor of Rheumatology, University of Leeds

The University of Leeds final examination in medicine
always has questions on the rheumatic diseases in the
written section, and patients with arthritic disorders
appear in the clinical assessment. This is true of virtually
every medical school in the country. Students will think of
few more cogent reasons for getting to grips with this
important subject. The emphasis in the exams is a
reflection of the importance in the community of these
disorders. They are the single most common cause of
morbidity in the population. In whichever branch of
medicine the doctor specialises rheumatic diseases are
prominent. The general practitioner will find that one in
four of the patients who call at his surgery have rheumatic
disease; the physician in a District General Hospital will
find a similar proportion of all medical referrals; the
radiologist will look with bleary eyes at the mountain of
bone and joint X-rays he has to report; the chemical
pathologist will find many metabolic abnormalities due to
rheumatic processes are reflected in his tests; the
immunologist will appreciate that rheumatology was the
subject that gave his discipline the biggest single boost;
the pathologist will often be asked to interpret specimens
from synovium, bone and other organs involved in diffuse
disorders of connective tissue; the microbiologist will find
that organisms both cause arthritis and are likely to infect
joints previously damaged by processes such as rheumatoid arthritis; and the community physician will scratch his
head to wonder how scarce resources can be stretched
to provide adequate care for the many rheumatic
sufferers in his district, and, if he has a conscience, in his
region.

For the teacher, rheumatic diseases provide one of the
best models for teaching medicine, as a Leading Article in

the British Medical Journal stressed.[1] Apart from the
principles of diagnosis and management which are
exemplified by rheumatic disorders, the sufferers frequently have physical signs that are important for the
student to recognise (in sharp contrast to many general
medical outpatients). It is imperative that at this stage he
grasps the fundamentals of the subject. Although
rheumatic diseases will play such a considerable part in
his future medical practice, he is unlikely to obtain more
postgraduate training in this area, however much he may
desire it.[2] This book has been written by two rheumato-
logists who have been engaged in busy practice, and who
have been associated with a Medical School that has long
recognised the importance of rheumatology in the
undergraduate curriculum. It will repay careful study both
in undergraduate and postgraduate days.

References

1. Leading Article (1979) Undergraduate education in rheumatology. *Br. Med. J.* **2**, 885–886.
2. Wright V. (1983) The consultant rheumatologist and postgraduate education. *Br. Med. J.* **287**, 1158–1159.

Soft-tissue rheumatism

The rather vague term, 'soft-tissue (non-articular) rheumatism', describes a multitude of painful conditions affecting the extra-articular soft tissues resulting from the trauma of everyday life. All are characterized by a self-limiting inflammation in the soft tissues, be they muscles, ligaments or tendons. Their incidence and chronicity increase with age. Many are well recognized and have a definite anatomical basis and treatment is usually straight-forward. These conditions are discussed in more detail below.

Other less specific 'aches and pains' occur but defy accurate anatomical diagnosis. These pains often emanate from muscle masses, particularly in the neck and shoulders, and are sometimes accompanied by tender, palpable nodules. The entirely spurious, though once popular term *fibrositis* is usually reserved for these ill-defined lesions despite the fact that no histological evidence of fibrous tissue inflammation can be identified. They usually respond to heat, soft-tissue massage and steroid injection. Mild non-steroidal anti-inflammatory drugs such as ibuprofen may be employed to good effect. The separation of these conditions from *psychogenic rheumatism* is often extremely difficult but failure to respond to adequate treatment in a clinical context of depression or anxiety should raise the suspicion that the patient is suffering from psychogenic rheumatism (*see below*).

The more easily identified conditions tend to occur around joints and as standard classification of these lesions tends to be cumbersome we have discussed the more common lesions in relationship to the joints around which they occur.

The shoulder joint

The shoulder joint is particularly vulnerable to soft-tissue lesions. This is probably because the joint has many planes of mobility and relies for its stability solely on the surrounding 'cuff' of muscles and tendons, any one of which can easily be damaged and give rise to 'the rotator cuff syndrome'. This is a rather vague term and a more accurate diagnosis should always be attempted.

◀ Soft-tissue lesions are common around the shoulder joint because it has many planes of mobility and relies for its stability on muscles and tendons.

Supraspinatus tendinitis. This is a very common problem. Patients complain of pain over the point of the shoulder often radiating into the root of the neck and over the deltoid region. Pain is made worse on movement, particularly abduction. Often the patient develops an arc of pain (*the painful arc*) when the shoulder is abducted and adducted (*Fig.* 1.1). This is a result of the tendon riding under the acromion and exacerbating the pain (*Fig.* 1.2). Occasionally it may develop into a chronic recurrent problem and deposition of calcium hydroxyapatite within the tendon occurs — *calcific tendinitis* (*Fig.* 1.3). Occasionally the tendon may rupture completely and the patient then has difficulty in initiating shoulder abduction.

◀ Supraspinatus tendinitis often produces a painful arc of pain on abduction of the shoulder.

Subacromial bursitis. The subacromial bursa (*see Fig.* 1.2) may become inflamed and give rise to exactly the same symptoms as supraspinatus tendinitis except that the pain is usually more constant and not so much influenced by the position of the

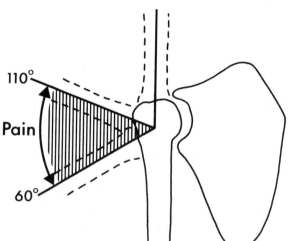

Fig. 1.1. Diagram showing the position of the 'painful arc' in supraspinatus tendinitis.

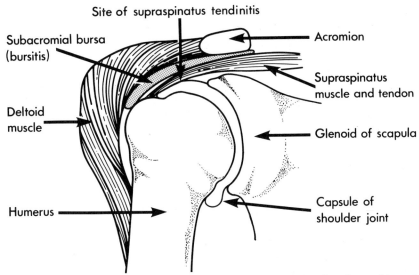

Site of supraspinatus tendinitis

Subacromial bursa (bursitis)

Deltoid muscle

Humerus

Acromion

Supraspinatus muscle and tendon

Glenoid of scapula

Capsule of shoulder joint

Fig. 1.2. Diagrammatic representation of the shoulder joint showing the position of the supraspinatus tendon and the subacromial bursa.

shoulder. It may be precipitated by crystal-induced inflammation within the bursa. As with supraspinatus tendinitis, tenderness can be elicited by deep palpation under the acromion at the point of the shoulder.

Treatment of both conditions with injection of local anaesthetic and steroid is usually curative, though recurrences are not uncommon. Early treatment is vital unless other structures around the shoulder joint are not to become involved and the patient develops a 'frozen shoulder' (*see below*).

Bicipital tendinitis. This is due to inflammation of the long head of biceps tendon within the bicipital groove. As the tendon emerges from the shoulder joint it is invested in a synovial sheath for a short distance and hence can be the site of synovitis in inflammatory arthritis, e.g. rheumatoid arthritis, but most cases are due to simple trauma. It is an extremely common condition and often mis-diagnosed. Pain around the anterior aspect of the shoulder joint may confuse the unwary into thinking its source lies within the joint itself but careful palpation will reveal that the maximum point of tenderness lies over the bicipital groove and that movements of the shoulder joint are full although external rotation may reproduce the pain as does

◄ Bicipital tendinitis gives rise to pain and tenderness over the anterolateral area of the shoulder and is often misdiagnosed as inflammation within the shoulder joint itself.

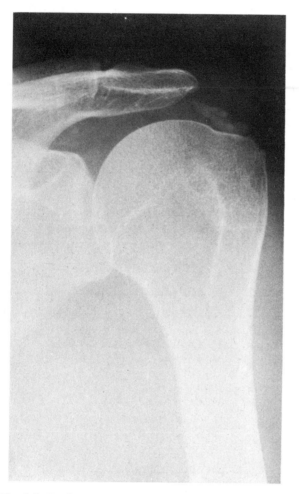

Fig. 1.3. Radiograph of a shoulder joint showing calcific tendinitis of the supraspinatus tendon. The patient, a young woman, presented with excruciating pain over the shoulder tip, and was unable to abduct her arm. Complete resolution was achieved within 48 h of a local steroid injection.

resisted flexion of the elbow. Injection of steroid into the immediate area around the tendon in the upper part of the bicipital groove over the maximum point of tenderness is usually curative. Ultrasound and local heat may also be helpful palliative measures.

'Frozen shoulder'. Any injury in and around the shoulder joint can result in a secondary loss of movement at the glenohumeral joint — the so-called

◀ The exact pathology of 'a frozen shoulder' is unknown. The term should only be reserved for conditions leading to *loss of movement* at the glenohumeral joint.

'frozen shoulder'. The exact pathology is uncertain but probably the capsule of the joint becomes inflamed and in some instances there may be a true synovitis of the joint resulting in the formation of fibrous adhesions within it. *Adhesive capsulitis* is another more explicit term for this condition. Any of the rotator cuff lesions can cause a secondary frozen shoulder, as can an inflammatory arthritis such as rheumatoid. It may also have an association with conditions which are far removed from the joint itself, such as myocardial infarction, pleurisy and hemiparesis. Referred pain pathways have been implicated in the first two conditions as causes of a frozen shoulder and in the case of hemiparesis the loss of supportive muscle tone around the joint may be responsible.

The patient complains of an inability to move the shoulder and often of a nagging pain centred over the joint and sometimes radiating into the deltoid area of the upper arm. Examination reveals loss of glenohumeral movement (*see* Chapter 14) and rotation is often painful. Tenderness over the anterior joint line may also be elicited.

◄ Inflammation within the shoulder joint may be referred to the deltoid area of the arm.

Prevention is the best form of treatment. This means treating all conditions likely to result in a frozen shoulder vigorously. Patients who have sustained a myocardial infarction should be encouraged to keep their shoulders mobile. The paretic arm of stroke patients should be passively moved regularly, and adequate sling support given. Once the condition is established treatment is extremely difficult. Intra-articular steroid injections should be given early followed by active physiotherapy. Manipulation of the shoulder may be undertaken very cautiously in resistant cases but is definitely contraindicated in patients in whom the joint itself is damaged, e.g. rheumatoid arthritis. In the majority of the more benign cases spontaneous resolution occurs but may take up to 18 months.

◄ Resolution of frozen shoulder may take 18 months or more.

The elbow joint

Medial and lateral epicondylitis (also known as golfer's and tennis elbow respectively). These conditions are extremely common and arise from inflammation around the tendinous origin of the wrist extensors (lateral epicondyle) and flexors (medial epicondyle). They are often precipitated by overuse of these muscles and patients experience severe pain and tenderness over the medial or lateral aspect of the elbow which can radiate into the forearm and occasionally into the upper arm. Pain can be made worse on resisted extension (in tennis elbow) or flexion (in golfer's elbow) of the wrist. Tenderness is usually elicited in a point distribution over the offending epicondyle. Treatment is by injection of local anaesthetic and steroid which in the majority of cases is curative although recurrences are common. Other forms of treatment such as ultrasound, heat and even binding the forearm muscles can sometimes give relief, though the majority of patients eventually settle spontaneously. A small minority may require surgical intervention before the condition resolves. Occasionally inflammatory arthritis, e.g. rheumatoid, may present as recurrent epicondylitis.

◀ Inflammatory arthritis, e.g. rheumatoid, may occasionally present as recurrent epicondylitis ('tennis elbow, golfer's elbow').

Olecranon bursitis. The olecranon bursa lies between the skin and the olecranon at the point of the elbow. Its function, in common with other subcutaneous bursae, is to allow free movement of the skin over a bony prominence. It can become inflamed and occasionally infected. Nodules may develop within it in rheumatoid arthritis. In gout urate deposition with secondary inflammation and tophi formation occur.

The wrist joint

Ganglia. These are usually hard cystic swellings found in association with joint capsules and tendons. They are particularly common around the wrist joint and usually present as a spontaneous swelling and are probably related to trauma. They are filled with hyaluronic acid and have a tough fibrous outer sheath which is contiguous with a joint capsule or tendon sheath. Often they can be dispersed by firm pressure but may disappear spontaneously. They are usually found over the extensor aspect of the wrists but sometimes in association with the flexor tendons of the fingers. Occasionally if they are painful surgical removal is recommended.

◀ Ganglia are found in association with joint capsules and tendons and are particularly common around the wrist joint.

De Quervain's tenosynovitis. This is caused by synovitis of the tendon sheath(s) of the abductor pollicis longus and/or extensor pollicis brevis at the wrist. The patient experiences severe pain on extension of the thumb or movement of the wrist, particularly ulnar deviation. The condition is invariably related to trauma and is more common in women. Tenderness is classically elicited over the tendons in the anatomical snuffbox. The pain may be reproduced by the patient making a fist around the thumb and the examiner forcing the wrist into ulnar deviation, thus stretching the inflamed tendons. Treatment is by infiltration of local anaesthetic and steroid, and resting the wrist in a suitable splint. The condition invariably settles without sequelae.

◀ In De Quervain's tenosynovitis tenderness is elicited over the extensor tendons in the anatomical snuffbox.

Carpal tunnel syndrome. Compression of the median nerve as it passes under the flexor retinaculum at the wrist produces characteristic symptoms of numbness and tingling in a median nerve distribution in the hand. If the condition is severe enough neurological weakness and wasting occur which are particularly noticeable in the muscles of the thenar eminence. The causes of this syndrome are:
1. So-called 'idiopathic' (probably representing a group of patients who have a congenitally shallow carpus and in whom the median nerve is therefore particularly vulnerable).
2. Arthritis of the wrist. It is sometimes a presenting feature of rheumatoid disease (*see* Chapter 5).
3. Fluid retention from whatever cause.
4. Hypothyroidism
5. Amyloid infiltration } less common causes.

Typically the patient awakes at night with tingling in the hand and pain extending into the forearm which is relieved by elevating the arm and shaking the wrist to assist venous return and effectively decompressing the carpal tunnel. Treatment in the first instance should be by a provision of a resting splint and the use of a mild diuretic. Many patients are cured by these simple measures but others require steroid injection beneath the retinaculum and some require surgical decompression.

◀ Carpal tunnel symptoms often wake the patient at night.

The hip joint

Trochanteric bursitis. This bursa lies between the insertion of gluteus maximus and tensor fascia lata and the greater trochanter of the femur. It not infrequently becomes inflamed and pain is localized to the upper outer aspect of the thigh but may extend downwards and is made worse by movement of the hip, particularly abduction. Tenderness over the greater trochanter can be easily elicited but movements of the hip joint are normal. Infiltration of the tender area with a local anaesthetic relieves symptoms immediately and a more lasting effect may be achieved by the injection of steroids.

Iliopectineal bursitis. Inflammation in this bursa which lies between the inguinal ligament and the iliopsoas muscle gives rise to pain in the anterior aspect of the hip (groin) and is exacerbated by hip extension. Tenderness is elicited just below the midpoint of the inguinal ligament and pain may extend into the anterior aspect of the thigh. It can be mistaken for intra-articular pathology of the hip joint but movements of the joint are full, though extension may be limited by pain. Again abolition of pain by infiltrating local anaesthetic can be diagnostic, steroid injections providing more long lasting relief.

Adductor tendinitis. This is an extremely distressing condition. Pain and tenderness are felt around the pubic tubercle radiating into the thigh. Resisted adduction of the hip is very painful and point tenderness may be elicited over the tubercle. Prompt relief is afforded by infiltration of local anaesthetic and steroid. This particular condition is common in athletic individuals and is not an infrequent cause of the so-called 'groin strain'.

Meralgia paraesthetica. Entrapment of the lateral cutaneous nerve of thigh beneath the inguinal ligament causes numbness and paraesthesiae in the lateral aspect of the thigh. Although symptoms are usually trivial, they can be extremely worrying for patients who may fear they are suffering from a more generalized neurological disease. The condition is particularly common in obese patients and also occurs as a complication of pregnancy. Dietary advice, the use of diuretics and occasionally infiltration of steroid around the nerve all provide symptomatic relief. Surgical decompression is necessary in only a few intractable cases.

◄ Meralgia paraesthetica (entrapment of the lateral cutaneous nerve of thigh) occurs in pregnancy and obese individuals.

The knee joint
Suprapatellar, prepatellar and infrapatellar bursitis (commonly known as 'housemaid's knee'). These conditions can give rise to considerable swelling over the anterior aspect of the knee and in the case of prepatellar bursitis obliterates the margins of the patella. Loss of the patellar contour is an important

sign in distinguishing patellar bursitis from an effusion within the knee joint itself. Aspiration of the fluid from the bursa and injection with steroids is the treatment of choice. Because of their superficial position the bursae may become infected.

◀ Supra- and prepatellar bursae may become infected.

Baker's cyst (popliteal cyst). This is a synovial pouch herniating from the knee joint into the popliteal fossa causing swelling and often interfering with flexion of the knee joint. The most common cause seen today is rheumatoid arthritis, but it may also occur in osteoarthritis. The cyst can become very tense due to synovial fluid being pumped into it from the knee joint and a valve-like mechanism at the neck of the cyst prevents the fluid from returning to the joint cavity. Not infrequently rupture of the cyst occurs and synovial fluid seeps into the calf muscles causing sudden intense pain and signs mimicking those of a deep venous thrombosis. The cyst can become very large indeed and track down the calf as far as the ankle. Aspiration of the knee joint often fails to disperse the cyst because of the non-return valve effect. Direct aspiration of the cyst is hazardous as a synovial leak may result with consequent pain, and infection is a real danger. Surgical removal and tying off the neck of the cyst, if it can be identified, is often difficult. Many cysts will eventually resolve and are in general best left alone provided symptoms from them are not too great.

◀ Symptoms of a ruptured Baker's cyst mimic those of deep venous thrombosis.

Semimembranosus and semitendinosus bursitis. A bursa between the tendons of semimembranosus and semitendinosus and the posterior aspect of the medial condyle of the tibia can become inflamed as a result of trauma ('pulled hamstrings') or synovitis in the knee joint itself with which the bursa communicates. Tenderness is elicited by deep palpation over the medial tibial condyle posteriorly. Aspiration and injection with steroid is the treatment of choice.

Quadriceps and calf muscle rupture. Rupture of a normal quadriceps muscle requires considerable force and the majority of ruptures are only partial and occur more commonly in muscles that are wasted as a result of knee joint arthritis. Pain is of sudden onset and can be intense. Examination may reveal a ridge of bunched muscle fibres in the anterior aspect of the thigh. Extension of the knee will be weak and if the quadriceps tendon has been ruptured will be lost completely. Treatment is by immobilization in a plaster-of-Paris cylinder for 3 weeks followed by physiotherapy. If the tendon is ruptured, early primary suture is vital if quadriceps function is to be maintained. Rupture of the calf muscles (again usually partial) occurs when the foot is forcibly dorsiflexed. Pain is of sudden onset and the calf can become severely swollen and tender due to the extravasation of blood forming a haematoma. A characteristic sign of this injury is a bruise occurring at the ankle a few days later.

◀ A characteristic sign of rupture of the calf muscles is a bruise occurring over the ankle a few days after the original injury. This condition may also mimic venous thrombosis of the calf.

Rest and the wearing of a suitable support stocking is usually the only treatment required. Because the signs of this condition mimic deep venous thrombosis of the calf, these patients are sometimes anticoagulated in error. This only serves to increase the size of the haematoma. A careful history is usually all that is required to differentiate the two conditions, though occasionally venography is indicated.

The ankle joint and foot

Achilles tendinitis. Inflammation around the Achilles tendon and its insertion into the posterior aspect of the calcaneum is most commonly caused by trauma, but also occurs in various arthritides, particularly those of the seronegative group (*see* Chapter 7). Pain may be severely disabling and cause the patient to limp. It usually extends from the heel, up the line of the tendon into the calf and a similar area of tenderness may also be elicited accompanied by some swelling. Point tenderness over the calcaneum usually indicates *Achilles bursitis*. Rest, heat and anti-inflammatory drugs may be used as a first line of treatment but rapid resolution is usually achieved by infiltration of steroid and local anaesthetic around (not into) the tendon. Advice about modifying shoes and the wearing of a protective pad may also be appropriate and a course of ultrasound for the more recalcitrant cases is often helpful.

Plantar fasciitis. The plantar fascia stretches from the anterior border of the calcaneum across the sole to the metatarsal heads. It becomes inflamed usually as a result of mechanical stresses. Pain is maximal over the inferior border of the calcaneum radiating into the sole and is exacerbated as the heel strikes the ground during walking and hence the patient tends to walk on his toes. It also occurs as part of a

◀ Recurrent attacks of Achilles tendinitis and plantar fasciitis in young males may be the presenting feature of seronegative arthritis. The most common cause, however, is trauma.

seronegative arthritis and indeed may be the presenting feature (*see* Chapter 7). Tenderness over the inferior border of the calcaneum (the heel pad) is often exquisite and sometimes extends along the fascia to the middle of the sole. Treatment is exactly as described for Achilles tendinitis. Shock-absorbing heel pads and insoles and modification of footwear help minimize symptoms and prevent recurrences.

Tarsal tunnel syndrome. Tarsal tunnel syndrome is analogous to carpal tunnel syndrome at the wrist. The nerve involved is the posterior tibial as it passes beneath the flexor retinaculum between the medial malleolus and the calcaneum. Symptoms of numbness and paraesthesiae in the sole occur and are usually relieved by infiltration with steroids. Occasionally surgical decompression is necessary.

Morton's metatarsalgia. Morton's metatarsalgia occurs as a result of a neuroma forming on an interdigital nerve usually of the second, third or fourth toe. It lies between two metatarsal heads and is therefore subjected to pressure causing lancinating 'electric shock-like' pain, radiating into the affected toes and back into the sole and occasionally up into the calf. Direct pressure over the toe web, either exerted from the sole or dorsally, will produce the symptoms, as will squeezing the metatarsal heads together. The neuroma may develop *de novo* or more usually as a result of forefoot arthritis, e.g. rheumatoid. Infiltration of the nerve with local anaeshetic will abolish the symptoms and is used as a diagnostic test. More permanent relief is achieved by surgical ablation. Steroid injection is also effective.

Psychogenic rheumatism

Minor musculoskeletal aches and pains are suffered by everybody at some time or other. Some patients, however, for some reason, e.g. emotional upset, depression, hypochondriacal or anxiety neurosis, develop a 'low pain threshold'. These everyday aches and pains then assume an intensity out of all proportion to their pathological significance. It is important to exclude other organic causes of pain before resorting to a diagnosis of psychogenic soft-tissue rheumatism. Once such organic disease

◄ Psychogenic rheumatism is a diagnosis which should only be resorted to after other organic causes of musculoskeletal pain have been ruled out.

has been ruled out it is vitally important to reassure patients that there is nothing seriously wrong with them as some patients in this group often have a morbid fear of crippling arthritis. In others their 'rheumatism' is an oblique way of bringing to the attention of a physician other, usually psychological, problems. If after a frank discussion of their symptoms the problem persists, social and psychiatric counselling may be required (*see* Psychogenic Back Pain in Chapter 3).

Osteoarthritis (Osteoarthrosis)   **2**

Osteoarthritis (OA) is a disease of the articular cartilage. It is extremely common and shows an increasing prevalence with age. Radiological evidence of OA, not necessarily symptomatic, is found in virtually all elderly people. The sex ratio is equal. Traditionally, OA is divided into two main groups:
1. Primary OA, i.e. no specific definable cause. This is the more common.
2. Secondary OA where a predisposing cause exists (*Table* 2.1).

Table 2.1.   Causes of secondary osteoarthritis

Trauma
  Malaligned fractures
  Excessive 'wear and tear'
    e.g. OA knees in coalminers
      Obesity
      Long leg arthropathy
      Old rickets

'Orthopaedic' conditions
  Congenital dislocation of the hip
  Slipped upper femoral epiphysis
  Perthes' disease of hip
  Epiphyseal dysplasia

Hormonal and metabolic causes
  Acromegaly
  Alkaptonuria (ochronosis) — deposition of homogentisic acid in hyaline cartilage, and subsequent calcium crystal deposition (i.e. chondrocalcinosis)
  Pseudogout
  Gout
  Kashin–Beck disease (due to ingestion of wheat contaminated with fungus, leads to premature OA. Seen in Eastern Europe)

The term *osteoarthritis* should really only be applied to cases in which there is definite evidence of joint inflammation (*see* Pathology) and not applied universally (though it often is!) as many cases have no inflammatory involvement when the term *osteoarthrosis* is to be preferred.

Aetiology

Surprisingly little is known about the causes of the cartilage damage in primary OA. Attrition due to ageing and prolonged use has for a long time been held responsible and given rise to the 'wear and tear' hypothesis (degenerative joint disease) and indeed there is much evidence to support this. A specimen of old cartilage is by no means as resilient as its younger counterpart and various subtle biochemical changes have been shown to take place as cartilage ages, such as loss of proteoglycans, increasing hydration and collagen fragmentation (*Fig.* 2.1). These changes in some measure help explain the lowered resilience — but this is not the whole story, and leaves unexplained the young patient with primary OA. There is ample evidence that excessive loads on a joint predispose to osteoarthritic changes within the cartilage. Such examples are the knees and elbow joints in coal miners and wrist joints in carpenters. However, when one looks at the distribution of osteoarthritis throughout the body,

◄ Excessive repetitive joint loading predisposes to OA.

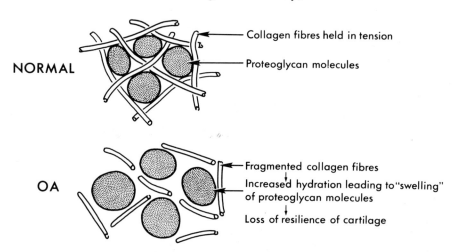

NORMAL
- Collagen fibres held in tension
- Proteoglycan molecules

OA
- Fragmented collagen fibres
- Increased hydration leading to "swelling" of proteoglycan molecules
- Loss of resilience of cartilage

Fig. 2.1. Diagrammatic representation of macromolecular changes occurring in osteo-arthritic cartilage.

one is struck by certain joints which are relatively free of OA but which undergo considerable load, e.g. ankles, shoulders. It should be noted that very little is known about the complex load factors acting through any joint in normal function and that many joints affected by OA which are regarded 'low load bearing', such as the distal interphalangeal joints of the hands and the sternoclavicular joints, may in fact at times be under considerable stress. How various stresses are transmitted through a joint is also ill-understood but clearly varies according to the *anatomical shape* of the joint and this may also be a factor in determining susceptibility to OA change.

Genetic factors have been implicated in primary OA but it is such a common disease that statistical analysis of any study is extremely difficult. There is some evidence that *Heberden's nodes* of the symmetrical variety (*see below*) are transmitted as an autosomal dominant trait with a reduced penetrance in males. The concept of *primary generalized OA* attempts to define a specific group of patients with *Heberden's nodes* and multiple joint involvement with a characteristic pattern of distribution, i.e. *proximal interphalangeal joints, posterior facet joints* of the *spine* and the *knees* with the hips, wrists and first metatarsophalangeal joints being less frequently affected. This particular pattern of OA is found in females over the age of 50.

◄ Primary Heberden's node positive, generalized OA is probably genetically determined. It is more common in females.

Although almost universal in an elderly population the extent of OA varies enormously between individuals, from clinically undetectable to extremely severe. Why some people should be more arthritic than others is yet another vexed question. Minor congenital abnormalities leading to loss of *joint congruity* (*Fig. 2.2*), particularly in the hip, have been suggested as an explanation for this, but evidence is lacking. In the final analysis *a multifactorial aetiology* will almost certainly have to be accepted.

◄ Loss of joint congruity predisposes to OA.

Pathology
The initial pathological changes take place in the articular cartilage. There is a gradual loss of stainable ground substance (proteoglycans) and a concomitant increase in hydration. Cellular proliferation occurs in the more superficial layers of the cartilage. The surface then splits and cracks with

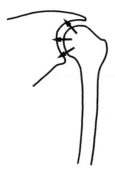 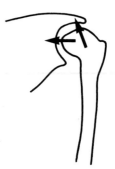

NORMAL JOINT
(good congruence of
articular surfaces)

ABNORMAL JOINT
(poor congruence of articular
surfaces leading to
maldistribution of load)

Fig. 2.2. Diagram illustrating the concept of loss of congruity of joint surfaces predisposing to OA change.

fissure formation (this is called *fibrillation*). At this stage acute synovial inflammation with a synovial effusion may occur giving rise to a true arthritis, but it is rarely as severe as that seen in rheumatoid disease and pannus formation is not a feature of OA, though villous hypertrophy of the synovium is sometimes seen. Cartilage is lost from the articular surfaces and there are sclerosis and remodelling of the subchondral bone with the formation of *osteophytes*. Bone cysts, formed by synovial fluid tracking down into the subchondral bone, are also a feature and are seen radiographically as lucent areas in the bone adjacent to the joint (*Fig.* 2.3).

◄ Pannus formation is not a feature of OA.

Clinical features

Symptomatology. Pain is the most common presenting complaint in OA. This can be severe and incapacitating. It is usually constant and made worse on activity and helped by rest of the affected joint. Acute exacerbations are not uncommon, especially in the knee, and these are often accompanied by signs of inflammation, i.e. warmth, tenderness and effusion.

◄ The pain of OA is made worse on activity and eased at rest.

The distribution of involved joints in OA is shown in *Fig.* 2.4. It will be noted that weight-bearing joints and the distal and proximal interphalangeal joints are commonly affected whilst the wrist, shoulders and ankles are less commonly involved. The arthritis

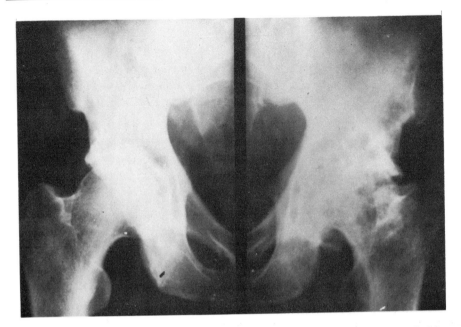

Fig. 2.3. Radiograph of osteoarthritic hip joint. *Note*, in the left hip: subchondral bone cysts; loss of cartilage (i.e. loss of 'joint space'); osteophyte formation; sclerosis of subchondral bone. (The right hip is normal.)

tends to be asymmetrical and often only affects one or two joints symptomatically though in most patients other asymptomatic joints can be detected on examination and even more radiographically. Early morning stiffness, such a common complaint in rheumatoid disease, is not a feature of osteoarthritis unless there is an inflammatory element present and even then it is shortlived. Transient *inactivity stiffness* of involved joints, however, is a feature. For details of the clinical aspect of *osteoarthritis of the spine* the reader is referred to Chapter 3.

◀ Joint distribution is *asymmetrical.*

◀ Early morning and inactivity stiffness may be a feature of OA if joint inflammation is present.

Examination findings
Examination of an involved peripheral joint might reveal the following features:
1. Nothing in early disease.
2. *Swelling* — This is due to either a *synovial effusion* (seen early or late in the disease) or a *bony swelling* (a feature seen in late disease due to bony remodelling). Posterior swelling of the knee joint called a *popliteal* or *Baker's cyst* is not

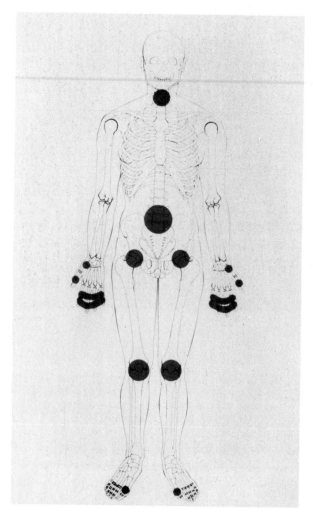

Fig. 2.4. Diagram illustrating distribution of osteoarthritis (*see* text for details).

uncommon and can occasionally rupture and give rise to symptoms and signs indistinguishable from deep vein thrombosis.

3. *Crepitus* — This results from cartilage damage and is easily palpable in affected joints, particularly the knee. Bony crepitus occurs in severely affected joints. It is sometimes audible. Crepitus can also originate from peri-articular structures, particularly the tendons of the rotator cuff at the shoulder (*see* Chapter 14).

4. *Limitation of movement* — This can be both passive and active limitation (*see* Chapter 14).

◄ Popliteal (Baker's) cysts may rupture and cause calf signs indistinguishable from deep vein thrombosis.

◄ Crepitus may arise from periarticular soft tissues as well as joints themselves.

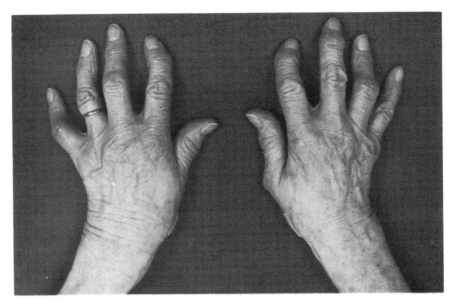

Fig. 2.5. Typical changes of OA of the hands, seen in a patient with osteoarthritis. *Note*: Heberden's nodes; Bouchard's nodes; subluxation of some joints; and 'squaring' of the left hand (*see* text for details).

5. *Deformity* — Joint deformities due to articular cartilage damage and bony remodelling are clearly seen in the hands, knees and feet.

In the *hands* the deformities are obvious. *Heberden's nodes* at the distal interphalangeal joints are sometimes associated with subluxation. *Bouchard's nodes* occur at the proximal interphalangeal joints. These nodes are made up of underlying outgrowths of bone (osteophytes) and cartilage from the lateral margins of the base of the distal and middle phalanx respectively (*Figs.* 2.5, 2.6). Damage to the first carpometacarpal joint causes loss of the lateral contour of the hand and results in a squared appearance (*Fig.* 2.5).

◄ Heberden's nodes occur at the DIP joints. Bouchard's nodes at the PIP joints.

Deformity of the *hip joint* can often be disguised by the patient, e.g. *adduction deformity* disguised by tilting the pelvis and flexing the contralateral knee. A *fixed flexion* deformity at the hip can often be missed on examination unless carefully looked for (*see* Chapter 14).

In the *knees* the most common deformities are:
a. Fixed flexion deformities.
b. Valgus (knock knees) and varus (bow legs)
Massive bony overgrowth of the femoral condyles

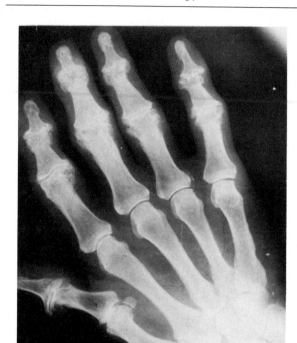

Fig. 2.6. Radiograph of hand of patient with OA. *Note*: osteophytes at base of distal phalanges (Heberden's nodes) and involvement of first carpometacarpal joint.

and upper end of the tibia can give rise to bizarre deformities.

Deformity of the first metatarsophalangeal joint resulting in *hallux valgus* ('bunions') is the most common sign of osteoarthritis involving the feet.

6. *Instability* — This is particularly common at the knee joint though by no means so common as in rheumatoid disease. The reason for this is that in OA bony remodelling with osteophytosis results in a relatively stable deformity whereas in rheumatoid arthritis there is often gross bone and cartilage loss and ligamentous damage and secondary muscle wasting, all key factors in maintaining joint stability.

7. *Signs of inflammation* — Acute, hot, painful swelling of osteoarthritic joints is not uncommon though inflammatory signs are not found as

◀ Joint instability results from:
bone and cartilage loss,
ligamentous damage,
secondary muscle wasting.

frequently as in rheumatoid arthritis. The majority of joint effusions seen in OA are found to be non-inflammatory on synovial fluid analysis (*see below*). OA joints can undergo recurrent inflammatory episodes and in this situation a careful search for *crystal deposition disease* must be made (*see* Chapter 8). As with any acutely inflamed joint, synovial fluid analysis is mandatory and must always include a full bacteriological analysis to rule out infection. Heberden's nodes can undergo episodic inflammation and become red and extremely painful. They may ulcerate.

◄ OA joints can become inflamed and crystal-induced synovitis may be the cause.

◄ Heberden's nodes can become inflamed and occasionally ulcerate.

8. *Disordered function* — Lower limb OA may cause the patient to *limp* and cause considerable disability, e.g. difficulty negotiating steps, getting up from a chair/toilet, etc. OA of the hands may cause problems with fine finger function as well as reducing grip strength.

Investigations
Osteoarthritis is a clinical diagnosis. The following investigations may be helpful in differentiating it from other arthritides in difficult cases:

1. Radiology
The characteristic radiological features of OA are:
a. Loss of the radiological joint space
b. Juxta-articular bony sclerosis and cyst formation
c. Osteophyte formation

} *See Fig. 2.3.*

It is important to remember that OA is a very common radiological finding and can coexist with other arthritides and radiological evidence of OA does not necessarily mean that OA is the cause of present symptomatology in any joint.

2. Laboratory investigations

ESR — This is invariably normal in osteoarthritis. If the ESR is persistently elevated then other causes must be sought. In this context polymyalgia rheumatica and multiple myeloma are important as they are more common in the elderly and it is this age group that is afflicted by OA. In inflammatory OA the ESR may be moderately elevated.

◄ The ESR may be moderately elevated in inflammatory OA.

Rheumatoid factor — This is not found in the serum of patients with OA and so helps differentiate them from patients with rheumatoid disease (*see* Chapter 5).

Synovial fluid analysis — OA synovial fluids are generally clear, viscous and straw coloured. The cell counts are low but occasionally during acute inflammatory episodes, the cell count can rise and often in these situations crystals of calcium pyrophosphate or hydroxyapatite can be found in the fluid (*see* Chapter 8).

◄ OA synovial fluid is viscous with a low cell count.

Treatment

The first aim of treatment is *pain relief*. Simple analgesic preparations such as paracetamol should be tried first. If these do not succeed, then an anti-inflammatory agent should be added. It is imperative that in addition to drug therapy, the patients are made aware of their condition and be prepared to modify their lifestyle accordingly. Thus the obese patient must *diet* and all patients should be taught the value of appropriate *exercises* by a physiotherapist to strengthen the various muscle groups acting on the affected joint.

Intra-articular injections of steroid preparations such as methyl prednisolone acetate and triamcinolone acetonide can be very effective provided the clinician is selective as to which joints to inject. Those with effusions and/or signs of active inflammation usually undergo a gratifying response to local steroid injection. Unfortunately such a response is often only shortlived but can give sufficient time for other measures, particularly physiotherapy, to be used with greater effect.

In some patients these conservative measures are insufficient to control their symptoms and their life is totally disrupted by their joint symptoms. It is in this group that joint *surgery* should be considered. The indications for joint surgery vary from patient to patient but *intractable pain*, marked *limitation of mobility*, and a failure to respond to all conservative measures are the three standard criteria used to assess a patient's suitability for surgery. There are many surgical procedures available for the relief of joint symptoms and their detailed discussion is outside the scope of this book. The reader is referred to a standard orthopaedic text for further information on this important topic.

Further Reading
Osteoarthrosis. In: *Clinics in Rheumatic Diseases*, December 1976. Philadelphia, Saunders.
Nuki G. (1979) *Aetiopathogenesis of Osteoarthrosis*. London, Pitman Medical.

Low back pain   3

Of all musculoskeletal complaints, backache is the most common. It has been estimated that at least 50% of people in the western world will suffer from back pain at some time in their life. Staggering statistics are often quoted to substantiate the enormity of the problem. Backache has been shown to cause more time off work than strikes in the United Kingdom and approximately one million patients consult their general practitioner with back-related problems each year. A third of these are subsequently referred to hospital clinics. Thus backache not only constitutes an enormous clinical problem but also a socioeconomic one. Much backache defies accurate diagnosis because its aetiology is usually obscure and in this chapter we can only give a broad overview of the subject.

◀ Backache causes more time off work than strikes in UK.

General principles

Anatomy
The spine is made up of a series of interlocking and articulating bones — *the vertebrae*. Each vertebra is separated from the next vertebra by a shock-absorbing cushion — *the intervertebral disc*. At its cephalic end the spine supports the skull and caudally, the pelvis. It comprises four reverse curves (*Fig.* 3.1):
a. Cervical
b. Thoracic
c. Lumbar
d. Sacrococcygeal

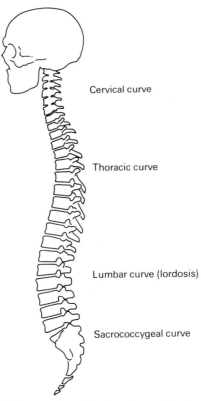

Cervical curve

Thoracic curve

Lumbar curve (lordosis)

Sacrococcygeal curve

Fig. 3.1. Diagram of vertebral column, showing the spinal curves.

Details of the articulations between each vertebra are shown in *Fig*. 3.2. The thoracic vertebrae have, in addition, articulations for the ribs (costovertebral joints). Each intervertebral disc forms a fibrocartilaginous union with the periosteum and bony end plates of the adjacent vertebral body. The apophyseal (posterior facet) joints are true synovial joints and allow for small amounts of gliding and rotational movements. Much of the load taken through the spine is transmitted via the vertebral bodies and intervertebral discs. The apophyseal joints are also load bearing, particularly in the lumbar spine. The whole structure is held as a stable unit by powerful ligaments and muscles. As well as providing a firm, yet flexible, pole onto which the rest of the skeleton is hung, the spine also functions as protection to the spinal cord and allows the nerve roots to pass via the intervertebral foramina.

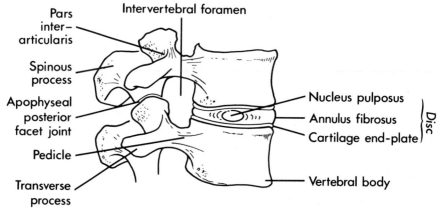

Fig. 3.2. Lateral view of two lumbar vertebrae showing the intervertebral articulations.

Spinal pain
The nerve supply of the various spinal structures and the appreciation of pain arising within them are not entirely understood.
1. The outer layers of the intervertebral discs receive a rich sensory innervation as does the periosteum of the vertebral bodies.
2. The capsule of the apophyseal joint also has a sensory innervation.
3. The dura of the spinal cord is another potential source of pain.
4. Pain can arise within vertebral ligaments and muscles if they are damaged in any way.

One of the greatest problems in assessing a patient with back pain is to determine from which particular structure the pain originates. In the majority of cases this does not matter in terms of treatment as most patients will be suffering from simple non-specific *mechanical pain* that is aggravated by motion and made better at rest. It often has a diffuse aching quality and can radiate into the buttocks and posterior aspects of the thighs. Whether such a pain arises from the apophyseal joints, the spinal ligaments or the paravertebral muscles, is immaterial, as most patients will settle by resting the spine by either bed rest and/or wearing a spinal support.

Pain that is not relieved by rest should always be regarded with suspicion as it may not have a simple mechanical cause. Constant *nagging* or *gnawing* pain unrelieved by rest or change of position and often waking the patient at night may be the indication of

◀ Mechanical back pain is relieved by rest. Pain not so relieved should be investigated thoroughly as it may have an inflammatory or malignant cause.

◀ Constant nagging or gnawing pain may indicate malignant disease.

bony pathology, e.g. *malignant deposits* or inflammation within the spine, i.e. *sacro-iliitis*.

Nerve root irritation from whatever cause gives rise to a characteristic sharp or shooting pain with radiation in a dermatome pattern down the leg(s). The nerve root may be compressed by a prolapsed disc, an osteophyte or any tumour obstructing the exit foramina, e.g. a neurofibroma.

Causes of back pain
Classification of the causes of back pain should help in making a rational diagnosis and such a classification is illustrated in *Table* 3.1. Many of these conditions are discussed elsewhere in this book.

Prolapsed intervertebral disc
This occurs as a result of the *nucleus pulposus* bursting through the *annulus fibrosus* of an intervertebral disc and causing pressure on surrounding structures (*see below*). It is often referred to in lay terms as 'a slipped disc' which is a totally misleading concept as the disc itself does not move. It may eventually become thinner due to loss of substance and this can be demonstrated radiologically. Any disc may prolapse but the most common are the *lumbar discs*, particularly those at L4/5 and L5/S1.

Aetiology
Each intervertebral disc comprises an outer tough, fibrocartilaginous ring (*annulus fibrosus*) surrounding the soft semi-fluid *nucleus pulposus* which is the embryological remnant of the notochord. The nucleus is made up of macromolecular complexes of mucopolysaccharides throughout which are scattered a few collagen fibres and fibroblasts. The design of the disc is ideally suited to its function as a shock absorber and it is this function which prevents shock waves from the lower limbs radiating through the pelvis, up the spine and into the skull.

As the disc ages the cellularity and fibrous content of the nucleus increases and its water content decreases. It thus becomes less elastic and therefore less able to absorb shock waves as they pass between the vertebral bodies. This loss of fluidity and

Table 3.1. Classification of back pain

The causes of back pain are given below although the list is intended to be an *aide-mémoire* rather than an exhaustive one.

Structural/mechanical back pain
Prolapsed intervertebral disc
. Spondylosis (degenerative joint disease of the spine), usually involving the apophyseal joints, often associated with degenerative changes of the intervertebral discs
Congenital abnormalities (usually scoliosis)
Spondylolisthesis (forward slip of one vertebral body on another), usually the result of degenerative disease in the adjacent lumbar disc and apophyseal joints, can also be congenital
Fractures (*a*) traumatic; (*b*) associated with metabolic bone disease resulting in thinning of the vertebral bodies; (*c*) invasion by metastatic tissue

Inflammatory
Ankylosing spondylitis
Spondylitis associated with psoriasis, inflammatory bowel disease or Reiter's syndrome
Scheuermann's disease (osteochondritis of the vertebral end plates)

Infectious
Tuberculosis
Brucellosis
Salmonella, resulting in vertebral osteomyelitis or paravertebral abscesses

Neoplastic
Almost invariably *metastatic*, the most common primary lesions being in the breast, bronchus, prostate, kidney, thyroid
Reticuloses and myelomatosis
Primary bone tumours

Benign tumours
Haemangiomas
Neurofibromata

Metabolic
Osteoporosis
Osteomalacia and renal osteodystrophy
Hyperparathyroidism
Ochronosis (alkaptonuria)

Paget's disease

Referred pain
Frequently of gynaecological origin in females
Renal disease
Pancreatitis or pancreatic neoplasm
Posterior duodenal ulcer
Abdominal aortic aneurysm

---

elasticity explains why herniation of the nucleus through the annulus fibrosus becomes less likely as the disc ages. The maximum incidence of prolapsed disc occurs in the third decade. Up to the second decade the disc structure is so strong that rupture of

◄ Disc prolapses tend to occur in the younger age group.

the annulus is very rare and requires considerable mechanical force.

The weakest part of the disc is the posterolateral region where the annulus is thinnest. Not surprisingly, most prolapsed intervertebral discs are seen in this area. This is a critical area where interference with nerve roots is most likely. However, prolapse can occur in other areas. Herniation of the nucleus pulposus posteriorly (*Fig.* 3.3) will cause direct pressure on the *postero-longitudinal ligament* of the spine and also on the *dura* which is extremely sensitive. If large enough, such a prolapse will encroach upon the spinal canal causing narrowing. This may jeopardize the descending nerve roots within the canal (particularly L5, S1 and S2) and lead to sphincter disturbances. This is a neurological emergency demanding urgent surgical referral. The combination of *perineal pain* and *numbness, flaccid paralysis* of the legs with *sphincter disturbances* resulting from such a posterior prolapse is known as the *cauda equina syndrome*. Other causes are vertebral body collapse, malignant deposits and local tumours.

It should be noted that enormous forces pass across the disc in everyday life but it is particularly susceptible to rotational and compressive forces. A prolapse may not necessarily be complete and the nucleus may only penetrate a few fibres of the annulus. This *partial prolapse* may give rise to pain without any root irritation.

◀ Most disc prolapses are posterolateral.

◀ Posterior disc prolapse may result in the cauda equina syndrome.

◀ Partial disc prolapse causes pain but not root irritation

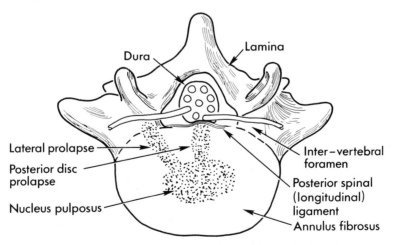

Fig. 3.3. A lumbar vertebra and disc showing the positions of a lateral and a posterior disc prolapse.

Clinical features

A classic presentation of a prolapsed intervertebral disc is of sudden onset of severe shooting pain in the back radiating down either leg in a dermatome distribution (*sciatica*). The pain is made worse on coughing or sneezing or any other manoeuvre that increases the pressure within the spinal canal. Radiation of the pain in a dermatome distribution is diagnostic of nerve root irritation. The nerve root(s) involved can be predicted from the particular dermatomes that are affected (*Fig.* 3.4). Nerve root pain often has a paraesthetic element to it, either burning or tingling, and may be associated with muscular weakness and later wasting.

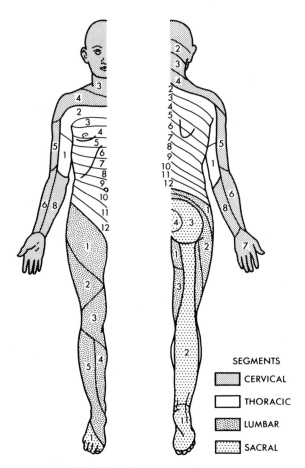

SEGMENTS

☐ CERVICAL

☐ THORACIC

☐ LUMBAR

☐ SACRAL

Fig. 3.4. The dermatomes.

Examination findings

In the acute stages the patient may be prostrate with *pain*, unable to move. Less severe cases adopt a posture of maximum comfort usually with a scoliosis and stoop and may well limp. Inspection of the spine confirms *scoliosis* convexed to the side of the prolapse. This is due to spasm of the paravertebral muscles. *Movements* of the spine may be severely restricted, the patient being extremely reluctant to move the spine in any direction less the severe pain be precipitated again. However, in general, lateral flexion of the spine is least affected whilst forward flexion is usually severely restricted. Rotation is also limited. Pressure over the relevant interspinous space may produce or exacerbate the pain. Straight leg raising (*see* Chapter 14) will be limited on the side of the root irritation. *Sensory changes* may be detected in a dermatome distribution (*Fig.* 3.4). Power should be tested by resisted hip flexion, knee flexion and extension, dorsiflexion and plantar flexion of the foot, inversion and eversion of the ankle, flexion and extension of the toes. *Reflex changes* may be transitory, the most commonly involved being the ankle, reflecting the fact that the L5/S1 disc is the most liable to prolapse.

◄ Disc prolapse results in severe spinal restriction and spasm of the paravertebral muscles.

◄ Forward flexion is severely limited, lateral flexion less so.

◄ The L5/S1 disc is the most common site of prolapse.

Investigations

Plain lumbar spine radiographs are usually unhelpful in the diagnosis of an acute prolapsed intervertebral disc. At most they will show and confirm the presence of a thoracolumbar scoliosis. Loss of disc height is not a sign of acute prolapsed disc but only indicates a disc that has undergone chronic degenerative change and as such is less likely to prolapse (*see above*).

Myelography using water-soluble contrast agents such as metrizamide is reserved for those patients in whom operative intervention is considered (*see* Treatment, *below*). It should be used to confirm the level of the prolapse. This will show either as an indentation in the opaque column of contrast within the spinal cord or as an interruption of flow down the affected nerve root sheath.

◄ Loss of disc height is not a sign of disc prolapse — it indicates chronic degenerative change.

Discography

During this procedure contrast medium is introduced into the disc itself using an image intensifier to guide the needle to the correct area. Injection of the contrast may often precipitate the patient's pain and escape of contrast out of the disc signifies a complete rupture of the annulus. It is a highly skilled technique and only available in a few centres and its value as a diagnostic aid in prolapsed discs has not yet been fully evaluated.

Treatment

1. Bed rest. This is by far the most important aspect of treatment of any disc prolapse. Provided there are no sphincter disturbances or rapidly progressive neurological signs the patient should rest supine on a firm bed. A board should be placed under the mattress if necessary or, failing that, the mattress placed on the floor if the bed does not give adequate support. Bed rest means just that, and the patient should only be allowed up to the toilet. Meals should also be taken with the patient lying as flat as possible. It is generally accepted that a trial of strict bed rest should last from between 4–6 weeks. If adequate bed rest cannot be guaranteed at home then the patient should be transferred to hospital.

◄ Complete bed rest is the mainstay of treatment of a prolapsed disc provided there are no advancing neurological signs.

2. Analgesia. In the acute stages, root and/or dural pain can be excruciating and demand opiate administration, e.g. pethidine 50–75 mg orally or i.m. given with a suitable anti-emetic. A useful analgesic and sedative combination is pentazocine and diazepam (50 mg pentazocine, 5–10 mg diazepam i.m.). When the acute stage has settled (usually 24–48h) analgesics may be switched to simpler agents such as distalgesic, paracetamol or dihydrocodeine.

3. Pelvic traction. The principle of applying traction to the pelvis is to distract the lumbar spine and relieve pressure on the offending disc and hence relieve pain. In practice a more important effect is to ensure that the patient stays still in bed. Many patients cannot tolerate pelvic traction and in some patients symptoms are made worse. Only a few will benefit but it is worth trying in some cases, particularly those who are not responding to simple bed rest, or who find it impossible to stay in bed.

4. Surgery. Removal of the fragments of the prolapsed disc by surgery (laminectomy) is indicated in those patients who:

a. Do not respond to adequate bed rest and in whom symptoms and neurological signs persist.

b. Patients with a central disc prolapse and sphincter disturbance (this is an absolute indication for surgical intervention).

If patients are selected on these criteria, the success of laminectomy is in excess of 80%. In patients with a longstanding PID results are less satisfactory.

5. *Post-acute treatment.* Once the acute pain has settled the patient is encouraged in gentle mobilization, gradually assuming the sitting position and eventually standing. During this rehabilitation period isometric abdominal muscle exercises are taught and, if necessary, the patient is fitted with a *lumbar corset support*, particularly if he or she has to resume work. This precaution ensures that the lumbar spine is not stressed unduly and patients learn to adapt their movements and avoid those which may cause relapse of their symptoms.

◀ Teaching patients how to protect their backs and adopt a correct posture is vital in preventing relapse of PID.

Degenerative spinal disease (spinal osteoarthritis)

This condition, as in osteoarthritis of the peripheral joints, is virtually universal in an ageing population. In many patients it gives rise to no symptoms and is detected by chance on pelvic or abdominal radiography. The radiological changes are characteristic and are termed '*spondylosis*'. It is important to note that lumbar spondylosis is not a clinical diagnosis, but a radiological one.

Aetiology

Changes of degenerative spinal disease are probably the result of ageing tissues being subjected to repeated minor trauma, i.e. wear and tear, in much the same way as degenerative disease occurs in the peripheral joints. It is not known exactly in which structures this degenerative process begins but it is very probable that *degeneration of the discs* is central to the whole process. As the discs age they lose resilience and their ability to resist impact shocks which are then transferred to the posterior joints and surrounding bone. Thus the cartilage of the posterior facet joints undergoes attrition and this process accelerates as it becomes older, just as

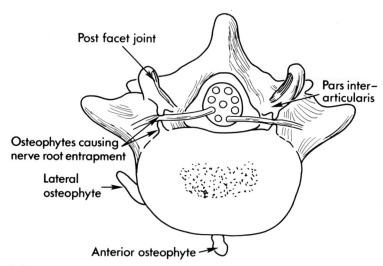

Post facet joint

Pars inter-
articularis

Osteophytes causing
nerve root entrapment

Lateral
osteophyte

Anterior osteophyte

Fig. 3.5. A lumbar vertebra showing the distribution of osteophytes seen in OA. *Note*: possibility of foraminal encroachment.

occurs in peripheral joint osteoarthritis with the formation of *osteophytes* (*Fig.* 3.5).

Clinical features

Pain of degenerative spinal disease tends to be of slow onset and diffuse. It is made worse on activity and eased at rest. It tends to be positional and a particular position, e.g. sitting for any length of time, may precipitate the pain. Conversely, a position such as lying on the side may relieve the pain. Acute exacerbations may occur on a background of chronic pain. These often follow minor trauma, such as twisting or bending, which may trigger an acute inflammatory synovitis of the posterior facet joints.

◄ Degenerative spinal disease pain is eased at rest and made worse on activity.

Examination of these patients is usually unrewarding, most signs being confined to alteration of posture. The lumbar lordosis is usually lost (this occurs progressively with age) and there may be *kyphosis* and *scoliosis* (*see* Chapter 14). Movements of the spine may be symmetrically reduced and tenderness may be elicited on percussion over the lumbar spine.

Symptomatic involvement of the *thoracic spine* resulting from degenerative joint disease is much less common than involvement of the lumbar spine, presumably because the forces acting through it are not as great. Osteoarthritis of the *costovertebral joints*, however, may cause symptoms which can lead to considerable diagnostic confusion. Posterior thoracic aching pain, made worse on breathing and sometimes having intercostal radiation due to involvement of the intercostal nerves as they emerge from the spinal canal, can mimic pleurisy. Pain on springing the ribs and localized tenderness over the costovertebral articulations are often useful discriminating signs.

◄ Osteoarthritis of the costovertebral joints may cause symptoms mimicking pleurisy.

Investigations

Radiography
As is the case in degenerative joint disease of the peripheral joints, the radiological incidence of degenerative joint disease of the spine increases with age. Thus degenerative joint disease seen on spinal radiographs, i.e. spondylosis, may not be the source of a particular patient's pain. The main function of radiographing a patient with suspected degenerative spinal disease is to rule out any other causes of back pain.

Changes associated with degenerative joint disease in the spine are (*Fig.* 3.6):
1. Loss of disc height.
2. Osteophyte formation at the junction of the discs and the vertebral bodies.
3. Sclerosis of the subchondral bone of the posterior facet joints.

Treatment
This can be considered under five headings.

Rest
As the pain of spinal degenerative disease is chronic then prolonged bed rest is clearly impractical. However, adequate rest can be provided for the lumbar spine by the wearing of a well-fitting support or corset. This method of treatment has the added advantage that patients whilst wearing them will be necessarily restricted and will learn how to adapt their pattern of movements so as to protect their already damaged lumbar spines. Fitting corsets to give adequate support to the thoracic spine is fortunately not often necessary but can be achieved.

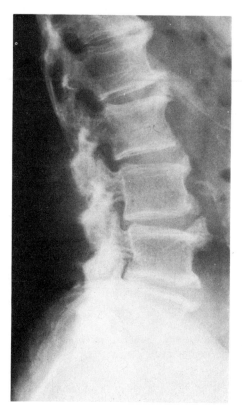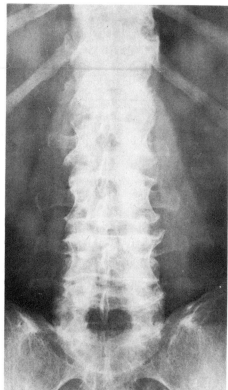

Fig. 3.6. Radiograph of lumbar spine showing degenerative joint disease. *Note*: osteophytes, loss of disc height and sclerosis of the posterior facet joints (apophyseal joints).

Active mobilization of the spine should only be performed by a trained physiotherapist and the hydrotherapy pool is probably the best area for this to be done. Specialized physiotherapy techniques such as *segmental mobilizing exercises* can be extremely beneficial.

Muscle strengthening exercises are often taught during the phase of active mobilization. Their place in the management of degenerative spinal arthritis is questionable. It is generally agreed that exercises which do not cause the patient any pain are harmless and may prevent further attacks.

Prevention
Educating patients in how to prevent or minimize their pain by such simple measures as posture

training, losing weight, teaching the correct way to lift and bend, is also extremely important.

Analgesia
Analgesia and/or anti-inflammatory medication should only be used as an adjunct to the treatment procedures mentioned above. It is important to stress to patients that drugs should only be resorted to when their pain is particularly severe. Simple analgesics such as paracetamol should suffice in the majority of patients. Many patients will also gain benefit from concurrent administration of short-term anti-inflammatory medication as many exacerbations of degenerative spinal pain have an inflammatory basis. Such non-steroidal anti-inflammatory drugs as aspirin, naproxen, indomethacin and azapropazone may be used in this context, though there are many more. Patient variability in terms of effectiveness of each individual drug is high, as is the incidence of side-effects (*see* Chapter 2).

Spondylolysis and spondylolisthesis
Spondylolysis is a defect in the *pars interarticularis* of a lumbar vertebra (*see* Figs. 3.2, 3.5). The defect is bridged by fibrous tissue and can be visualized on an oblique radiograph as a radiolucent zone. It was originally regarded as a congenital defect and indeed some cases probably are, but some cases are the result of inadequately healed *fatigue fractures*. The condition shows a strong hereditary influence.

Symptoms do not usually arise until the early teens and spondylolysis is an important cause of low back pain in this age group. If the defect is severe enough it will allow the affected vertebra to slip forward on the one below. It is this slip that is known as *spondylolisthesis*. Occasionally nerve entrapment may result. The most common vertebrae to be affected are L4/5 and L5/S1. The condition may not highlight itself until adulthood and a defect in the pars interarticularis is seen in the majority of these cases up to the age of 50. It may be an incidental finding on lumber spine radiography and not necessarily the source of symptoms; however, the younger the patient the more likely it is that spondylolisthesis is the cause of the symptoms.

◀ L4/5 and L5/S1 are the most common sites of spondylolysis.

The other form of spondylolisthesis is thought to be due to degenerative changes in the intervertebral disc and apophyseal joints which eventually place undue stresses on the pars interarticularis allowing a forward slip. This type of spondylolisthesis is known as *degenerative* or *'acquired' spondylolisthesis* and is seen more frequently in patients over the age of 50. Direct fracture of the pars interarticularis due to severe trauma is a rare cause of spondylolisthesis.

Treatment of the condition is extremely difficult. Most patients, however, will respond to a lesser or greater extent to a period of rest and then mobilization in a suitable lumbar-sacral support. More severe cases with neurological signs may require extensive surgery with a decompressing laminectomy and bone grafting to stabilize the spine.

Spinal stenosis

Narrowing of the lumbar spine canal (*stenosis*) can cause pressure of its contents and result in nerve root pain. This narrowing is usually the result of degenerative changes with osteophytes protruding into the canal superimposed on a congenitally narrow canal; thus incidence increases with age.

A characteristic symptom is *neurogenic claudication*. This comprises root pain, sensory changes in a dermatome distribution and muscle weakness which are typically precipitated on exercise and disappear at rest. The association of these symptoms with exercise is extremely important in making the diagnosis of spinal stenosis. It arises because the blood vessels supplying the nerve roots are compressed in the narrow canal and intervertebral foramina. Blood supply becomes compromised on exercise as it is diverted to muscles. It is important to differentiate neurogenic claudication from intermittent claudication caused by peripheral vascular disease which does not give rise to any nerve root symptoms. A further differentiating feature is that neurogenic claudication tends to take longer to ease at rest.

◀ Neurogenic claudication often has a paraesthetic element and takes longer to ease at rest than intermittent claudication.

Examination of the lower limbs at rest may be entirely normal, in particular peripheral pulses are all present (unless the patient has coexisting peripheral vascular disease). However, neurological examination after exercise may reveal sensory changes in a root distribution and/or muscle weakness and reflex changes such as loss of knee or ankle jerk which return after a suitable period of rest.

Ankylosing hyperostosis (Forestier's disease)
In this condition affecting older males, there is *gross osteophytosis* of the thoracolumbar spine resulting in *bony bridging* between vertebra. The thoracic spine is affected first in the majority of cases but it usually spreads to involve the upper lumbar spine. The fusing of adjacent osteophytes and the formation of bony bridges can give rise to radiological diagnostic confusion with ankylosing spondylitis. Points of differentiation are:
1. Older age of presentation.
2. No involvement of the sacro-iliac joints.
3. Distribution of spinal changes (the cervical spine is not involved).
4. The condition is rarely painful but does lead to progressive spinal stiffness.
It is sometimes detected coincidentally on radiographs of the chest or abdomen in patients who have no spinal symptoms.

Scheuermann's disease (osteochondritis of the spine)
This condition primarily affects the thoracic spine of *adolescent males*. It is often asymptomatic and only discovered on spinal radiographs later in life. These changes comprise an irregularity of the epiphyseal end plates of the vertebral bodies often with anteroposterior wedging and narrowing of the corresponding intervertebral disc. This results in a *smooth kyphosis*. When symptoms do arise, they consist of a dull ache over the lower thoracic spine and occasional intercostal radiation. They usually respond rapidly to anti-inflammatory medication. Care must be taken to distinguish these patients from those with ankylosing spondylitis as the prognosis in Scheuermann's disease is uniformly good as far as future spinal function is concerned.

Investigation of the patient with back pain
A full medical history and examination should be obtained in every patient presenting with back ache. Only in this way will those patients with underlying systemic disease be detected. The decision as to which patients with back pain should be investigated is an extremely important one. The number of

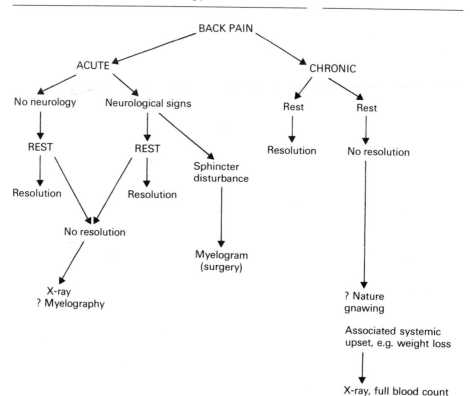

Fig. 3.7. Flow diagram illustrating guide lines for investigation of back pain.

patients presenting with back symptoms is enormous and the majority of these suffer simple mechanical pain which settles without medical intervention. The following flow diagram (*Fig.* 3.7) should act as an *aide-mémoire* in making the decision to investigate.

Psychogenic back pain

It is not surprising that back pain figures largely in the symptomatology of patients seeking attention because of a hidden psychological problem, usually of a depressive nature. It is sometimes very difficult to identify these patients and the situation is further complicated by the fact that objective evidence of back pathology is sometimes present on clinical examination (rarely) or radiologically (commonly). The social background or a previous history of

depression or psychotic episodes are vitally important clues in these patients. Reliance has to be placed on three factors:
1. History
2. Examination
3. Subsequent course of pain

History

In a patient with psychogenic back pain the history often gives clues as to the non-organic extent of the symptoms. Inability to localize pain to a particular area of the spine ('the pain all over' syndrome) is not uncommon in this group of patients. Inconsistencies in the history, particularly in the answering of such questions as 'is the pain worse at rest?' and 'do you get any relief on movement?' are also often elicited. Care must be exercised in the interpretation of these inconsistencies as patients often have a genuine inability to describe their back symptoms adequately. However, these patients usually respond in a meaningful way to leading questions. Persistently negative response to analgesia and/or anti-inflammatory drugs given in adequate dosage should be regarded with suspicion.

Examination

Careful and thorough examination of these patients is essential and often illuminating. A patient who claims to be incapacitated by pain and yet shows a full range of spinal movement (all be it with some encouragement) is clearly either over-reacting or has no organic symptoms at all. Such clearcut cases are not uncommon. A negative examination in the face of gross symptomatology is an important pointer, although not entirely foolproof. If limited spinal mobility is confirmed on direct examination of the spine it is often useful to observe the patient whilst dressing. He may well be able to bend quite easily to put on his socks and tie up his shoe laces whilst a few minutes before he was claiming that he was unable to flex his spine at all.

◄ A negative examination in the face of gross symptoms is a useful indication of psychogenic back pain.

Subsequent course of the pain

Psychogenic back pain often undergoes wild swings of severity without concomitant swings in the

number or degrees of objective physical signs. These
swings in symptomatology can often be related
directly to some triggering event in the patients'
social history. They may be clinically depressed. As
our knowledge of the various aetiological aspects of
back pain is somewhat incomplete, the diagnosis of
psychogenic back pain must, as in all cases of
psychosomatic disease, only be resorted to when all
other possibilities have been excluded.

◄ A diagnosis of
psychogenic back pain
must only be made when
no organic pathology can
be found.

It is important to make full assessment of patients
who are often extremely worried about their back
pain and its significance. Fear of malignant disease is
one of the most common in this regard. Having
established that there is no significant pathology in
their spine, the patients should be told that their
back pain is not serious and will not result in any
permanent disability. Many patients will be greatly
reassured by this approach but those who are not
and who continue with their psychogenic back
symptoms should be referred for social counselling
and possibly a psychiatric opinion.

Further Reading

Evans D.P. (1982) *Backache: its Evolution and Conservative Treatment.* Lancaster, MTP.

Waddell G. (1982) An approach to backache. *Br. J. Hosp. Med.* **28/3**, 182.

Cervical pain　　　　4

Neck pain is a common cause of patients seeking rheumatological advice. Degenerative joint disease is by far the most common cause of symptoms but disc lesions and secondary nerve root compression also occur. These and other causes of neck pain are shown in *Table* 4.1.

◄ Degenerative joint disease is the most common cause of neck pain.

Cervical spondylosis
Degenerative joint and disc disease of the cervical spine occurs in 60% of people over the age of 35 and the incidence increases with age as does osteoarthritis elsewhere in the skeleton. The joints involved are the apophyseal joints and the neurocentral joints. Distribution of arthritic changes shows a predominance in the lower cervical spine, but any level, often multiple, may be affected. As in lumbar spondylosis (*see* Chapter 3), degenerative disc and joint disease evolve together. Acute cervical disc lesions are not common and tend to occur in younger patients who have suffered trauma, e.g. whiplash injury or sudden violent twisting movements.

◄ Cervical spondylosis tends to affect the lower cervical spine.

Table 4.1.　Causes of neck pain

1. Degenerative joint disease (cervical spondylosis)
2. Rheumatoid arthritis
3. Ankylosing spondylitis
4. Cervical disc lesions
5. Referred pain, e.g. myocardial ischaemia, apical lung tumours (Pancoast)
6. Thoracic outlet syndromes (cervical rib, 'drop' shoulder, etc.)
7. Non-specific muscular pain, e.g. 'stiff neck'
8. Non-musculoskeletal, e.g. lymphadenitis

It is more common for such an injury to trigger chronic cervical pain with nerve root irritation in a patient who already has cervical spondylosis.

Clinical manifestations

Stiffness and *pain* in the neck often radiating into the shoulders and sometimes accompanied by headache are the typical presenting symptoms. Attacks may be frequent and interspersed with pain-free intervals. *Neurological manifestations* are common as osteophytosis causes foraminal and spinal canal encroachment. Paraesthesiae occur radiating down the arm in a dermatome distribution (*see Fig.* 3.4) corresponding to the affected nerve roots (*cervical radiculopathy*). Muscle weakness may also ensue, particularly in the hand. Neurological symptoms and neck pain often wake the patient from sleep. As the arthritis advances and osteophytosis increases, the vertebral arteries may become trapped, jeopardizing brainstem blood supply and resulting in transient ischaemic attacks particularly on hyperextension of the neck (so-called *drop attacks*). The spinal canal is at its narrowest in the cervical spine and may become even narrower and result in spinal cord compression. This can present insidiously as weakness and paraesthesiae in the legs and arms and urinary symptoms such as urgency and hesitancy. The clinical picture can be confusing as spinal root and cord compression may coexist giving rise to upper motor neurone signs in the legs and lower motor neurone signs in the arms. In view of the fact that cervical spondylosis affects the older age group, motor neurone disease is the chief differential diagnosis but the presence of sensory symptoms and signs makes a diagnosis of cervical spondylosis certain. As with patients with back pain, a thorough neurological examination is thus mandatory. Other neurological signs such as Horner's syndrome (due to pressure on the cervical sympathetic chain), nystagmus, cerebellar signs and hemiplegia (due to brainstem ischaemia) occur rarely.

◀ Neurological symptoms affecting the arms are common in cervical spondylosis.

◀ Pressure on the vertebral arteries by osteophytes can cause brainstem ischaemia and drop attacks.

◀ Sensory symptoms and signs occurring in cervical spondylosis help differentiate it from motor neurone disease.

Investigations

Radiographs of the neck show anterior and lateral osteophytes with loss of disc height and sclerosis of the apophyseal joints (*Fig.* 4.1).

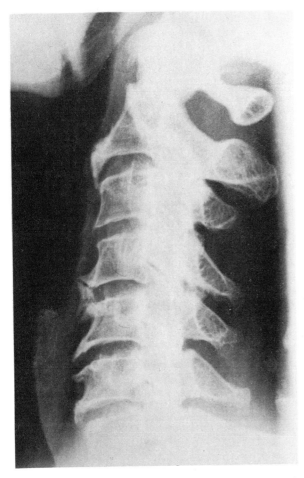

Fig. 4.1. Lateral radiograph of cervical spine showing osteophytes, disc space narrowing and sclerosis of apophyseal joints, i.e. degenerative joint disease or cervical spondylosis.

Treatment

Rest
This is by far the most important factor in any treatment regime for neck pain. It is best achieved by fitting the patient with a suitable collar and warning him that it may feel uncomfortable for a while before its full effect can be appreciated. Posture at night is also important and patients should be encouraged to sleep with one pillow. Many patients arrange their pillows to give maxi-

mum pain relief and comfort, e.g. rolling the pillow into the curve of the neck.

Analgesia
Mild analgesics may be used (e.g. paracetamol, codeine). In some patients non-steroidal anti-inflammatory drugs afford more relief presumably due to the fact that secondary inflammation as well as mechanical pain is present.

Physiotherapy
Traction may be of value especially in those patients with neurological symptoms. A quick test to assess whether traction will be of benefit is gently to distract the cervical spine vertically by pulling upwards under the angle of the jaw. If symptoms are relieved by this manoeuvre then a course of traction is indicated as it is if there is an increase in symptoms when the neck is compressed by firm downward pressure on the head. Heat and massage often give temporary soothing relief.

Thoracic outlet syndrome
The nerve roots C8 and T1 form the lower trunk of the brachial plexus which, with the subclavian artery and vein, passes behind the scaleneus anterior muscle and between the clavicle and first rib. In this position it may become compressed giving rise to paraesthesiae and pain down the medial aspect of the arm into the little finger and up into the axilla (C8 T1 dermatomes). Such symptoms are exacerbated by carrying heavy loads or when the shoulder girdle droops due to poor posture (*drop shoulder*). Occasionally a nerve trunk and subclavian artery become compressed by an extra rib articulating with C7 (*cervical rib*) or by the scaleneus anterior muscle. In addition to neurological symptoms patients may also experience vascular symptoms, e.g. cold, blue, swollen hand and even thromboembolic episodes due to damage of the vascular endothelium of the subclavian artery. A vascular bruit may be heard at the root of the neck and the brachial and radial pulses may be diminished. Classically, symptoms of a thoracic outlet syndrome are abolished by raising the arm above the head and patients often indulge in this manoeuvre to gain relief.

◄ The symptoms of thoracic outlet syndrome are often relieved by raising the affected arm above the head.

Treatment
Simple shoulder-raising exercises and the teaching of
correct posture are all that some patients require to
achieve symptomatic relief. In others where symptoms are more severe, exploration of the root of the
neck is required with division of the scaleneus
anterior or the removal of a cervical rib which in
many cases proves to be a vestigial fibrous cord,
invisible on radiography.

◄ Cervical ribs may be
invisible on radiography,
comprising only a vestigial
fibrous cord.

**Neuralgic amyotrophy (acute brachial neuritis,
brachial neuralgia)**
This condition is acute and self-limiting and is
thought to be the result of a viral infection although
it has been described following serum sickness. The
cervical as well as the brachial plexus may be
involved. It is usually symmetrical in distribution,
although not in intensity. The patient complains of
severe pain and paraesthesiae radiating from the
shoulder down the arm into the hand. Muscle
tenderness and weakness over the shoulder, neck
and arm also occur. Objective signs are of diminished reflexes and sensory impairment. Rest and
analgesia are all that are required and the severe
pain usually settles within days with complete
resolution over 2 months. Occasionally recovery
may take longer if there has been extensive
neurological damage. Some patients are left with
permanent disability around the shoulder girdle.

Further Reading
Jeffreys E. (1980) *Disorders of the Cervical Spine*.
London, Butterworths.

Rheumatoid arthritis   5

Rheumatoid arthritis (RA) is an inflammatory disease of synovial membranes, usually presenting as a polyarthritis, which can have far-reaching systemic manifestations. It is a common condition and has a worldwide distribution but it is more prevalent in temperate climates. It affects approximately one-and-a-half million people in the UK, 6% being females and 2% males. The majority of patients have their first symptoms between the ages of 20 and 55 years, but the age range extends from 16 years to 70+ years. Children are also affected by a disease indistinguishable from adult rheumatoid arthritis (*see* Chapter 12).

◀ Rheumatoid arthritis is primarily a disease of synovial membranes.

Pathology
In RA the synovial membrane becomes inflamed and proliferates, forming villi which encroach upon the 'joint space'. This characteristic inflammatory tissue containing numerous polymorphs, lymphocytes and plasma cells is highly vascular and has the histological characteristics of granulation tissue, and is called *pannus*. At points of contact between pannus and hyaline cartilage, proteolytic enzymes are released and digest the cartilage, and the pannus is thus able to burrow into the articular cartilage and subchondral bone giving rise to the pathognomonic bony erosion seen radiographically. This process starts at the outer margins of the joint but gradually spreads across the articular surface. The resultant loss of articular cartilage, and the damage to the subchondral bone are prime factors leading to the

◀ Synovial pannus formation is characteristic of rheumatoid synovitis.

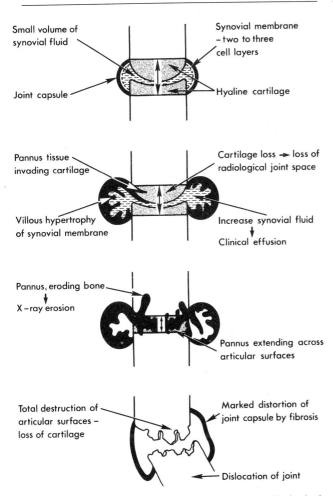

Small volume of synovial fluid

Synovial membrane – two to three cell layers

Joint capsule

Hyaline cartilage

Pannus tissue invading cartilage

Cartilage loss ➤ loss of radiological joint space

Villous hypertrophy of synovial membrane

Increase synovial fluid
↓
Clinical effusion

Pannus, eroding bone
↓
X – ray erosion

Pannus extending across articular surfaces

Total destruction of articular surfaces – loss of cartilage

Marked distortion of joint capsule by fibrosis

Dislocation of joint

Fig. 5.1. Diagrammatic representation of pathological joint changes occurring during the course of rheumatoid arthritis.

disruption of the joint. Hyaline cartilage has a very limited power of regeneration and healing is by fibrosis. In later stages of the disease the fine histological detail of the synovial membrane is totally lost and is replaced by fibrous tissue which causes contracture of the joint capsule and adds to the general destructive process (*Fig.* 5.1).

Any synovial tissue can be affected by this process and that contained in tendon sheaths, particularly in the hands, is no exception, and is often a contributory factor to the hand deformities seen in the disease.

◀ Hyaline cartilage has limited powers of regeneration.

◀ Any synovial tissue may be involved in RA including tendon sheaths.

Synovial fluid changes

In a normal joint very little synovial fluid is present. It is clear and viscous with a very low coefficient of friction. It forms a lubricating film between the articular surfaces of the joint. In response to the inflammatory process of rheumatoid arthritis the synovium secretes increased amounts of synovial fluid resulting in a joint effusion. This fluid is thin and contains high concentrations of proteolytic enzymes which degrade the macromolecular complexes of mucopolysaccharides that give the fluid its normal viscous characteristics. It also has a high cell content, the predominant cell being the polymorph, and this accounts for the increased turbidity of the fluid macroscopically. Occasionally the cell content can be so high as to give the appearance of pus to the synovial fluid but the fluid is sterile on culture.

The pathology of the various extra-articular features are discussed briefly under their separate headings in the clinical section.

◀ Synovial fluid cell content may be so high as to give the appearance of pus.

Aetiology

The cause of rheumatoid arthritis is still unknown despite intense and dedicated research. It is impossible here to discuss all the current aetiological concepts of the disease but any hypothesis has to explain the following facts:

1. The primary target organ is the synovium.
2. The chronicity of the disease.
3. The various immunological disturbances that occur during the disease.

For a long time some form of infection was thought to be responsible and led to diligent searching for an infective agent. Diphtheroid bacilli and mycoplasmas have both been implicated only to be rejected on the grounds that they are not consistently found in the joints or the blood of patients, even in early disease. The possibility that the inciting agent is a virus, or viruses, is an attractive one, as a virus or parts of a virus are capable of incorporation into the nuclei of cells and thus resist detection. There is some evidence that synovial cells in patients with RA are infected with a virus, but again evidence is not sufficiently strong to implicate a particular virus. The other attraction of the viral theory is that viral particles incorporated into the synovial cell would be capable of providing either directly or indirectly (by programming the synthesis of a specific protein) the *chronic antigenic stimulation* thought to be necessary for sustaining synovial inflammation.

The concept of a 'hidden antigen' fuelling the disease process in a genetically predisposed individual serves as the basis for much present-day research. An example of this predisposition would be the recent discovery that a specific genetically-determined tissue antigen (HLA DR4) carried on B-lymphocytes is found in increased frequency in patients with rheumatoid arthritis. The association of this particular antigen and rheumatoid disease is, however, by no means as strong as the association of the histocompatibility antigen HLA B27 and ankylosing spondylitis (*see* Chapter 7), but at least gives some credence to the idea that certain individuals are predisposed to rheumatoid disease. Family studies of patients with RA, however, give no clear pattern of inheritance in the disease though a strong family history of the disease is by no means uncommon.

The concept that RA is an 'autoimmune' disease and that the underlying disorder is an abnormal immune reaction directed against 'self' antigens that may or may not have been altered by some external agent, is an attempt to explain the chronicity and the obvious immune disturbances that occur in the disease. However, it is now widely held that the immune disturbances seen in RA, such as the synthesis of antiglobulins (rheumatoid factors – *see* Laboratory investigations), infiltration of tissues with lymphocytes and plasma cells, and susceptibility of RA patients to infections, are all probably secondary phenomena to some other central aetiological factor.

Other aetiological hypotheses, such as altered nutrition, inborn errors of metabolism, an endocrine abnormality, occupational factors and climatic factors (damp and cold), have not withstood the critical appraisal of various epidemiological surveys.

Clinical features

Early

The majority of patients have an insidious onset of symmetrical joint pain, stiffness and swelling, worse

◀ Onset usually insidious.

in the early morning and usually starting in the hands, wrists and feet. The classic patient is a female in her third decade who may already have experienced several episodes of such joint pain before seeing her practitioner, the visit being precipitated by more prolonged or more frequent attacks and a feeling of general malaise. About 15% of patients present acutely with a debilitating symmetrical joint inflammation, often involving numerous joints but invariably the metacarpophalangeal (MCP) and the proximal interphalangeal joints (PIP) in the hands, and the metatarsophalangeal (MTP) joints in the feet. These patients can be extremely ill, undergo rapid weight loss, swinging fever and night sweats.

◀ Typically affects young females.

◀ 15% of cases present acutely.

Monoarthritis, usually of a knee, sometimes of a shoulder or ankle, can be a presenting feature and can give rise to difficulty in diagnosis, the differential diagnosis being trauma, sepsis, seronegative arthritis (*see* Chapter 7), or crystal-induced arthritis (*see* Chapter 8). If, however, such patients are followed up closely, eventually all will develop the more typical symmetrical small joint involvement of rheumatoid arthritis.

The cardinal points in making a clinical diagnosis of rheumatoid arthritis are summarized below:
1. Clinical evidence of synovitis.
2. Distribution of such synovitis — symmetrical and primarily involving the MCP and PIP joints, the wrists and the MTP joints.
3. Early morning pain and stiffness in the involved joints which can be 'worked off' as the day progresses — this is particularly true of the hands.
4. A relapsing and remitting course.

Established disease
As the disease progresses and the joint damage increases, characteristic deformities develop.

The hands
At the *metacarpophalangeal* joints there is ulnar deviation and the joints eventually dislocate (subluxation) (*Fig.* 5.2). Swan neck and boutonnière (*Fig.* 5.3) deformities occur at the interphalangeal joints.

◀ MCP and PIP joint involvement occurs. Ulnar deviation at the MCP joints is characteristic.

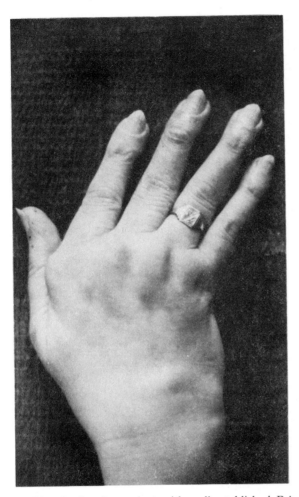

Fig. 5.2. Hands of a patient with well-established RA. Note ulnar deviation at MCPs and prominent ulnar styloid process.

The wrists

The wrists become swollen, particularly over the extensor aspects, and the ulnar styloid processes become prominent, tender and can be 'sprung' up and down with pressure, indicating involvement of the inferior radio-ulnar joint and destruction of the annular ligament. Inflammation within the extensor tendon sheaths and stretching of the tendons over a distended wrist joint or dislocated ulnar styloid can cause tendon rupture resulting in the sudden inability to extend a finger ('*dropped*' *finger*).

◄ Dislocation of the inferior radio-ulnar joint and a 'sprung' ulnar styloid are common findings in a rheumatoid wrist.

a

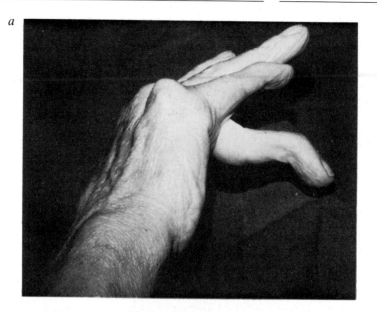

b

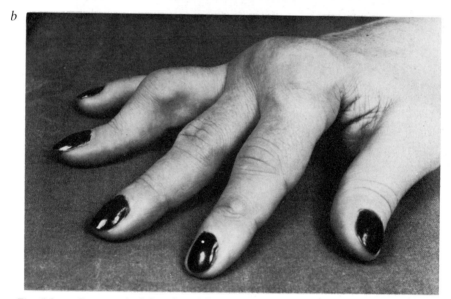

Fig. 5.3. *a*, Swan neck deformity of finger. *b*, Boutonnière deformity of ring finger.

The elbow joint

Involvement of the elbow joint usually causes considerable pain and functional disability. Fixed flexion deformities at this joint are not uncommon. The superior radio-ulnar joint is commonly involved and causes pain on supination and pronation of the forearm and tenderness and crepitus can be elicited over the joint line below the lateral epicondyle.

The shoulders
The shoulders show loss of motion and sometimes anterior swelling with tenderness denoting an acute synovitis with effusion. A young patient presenting with bilateral 'frozen' shoulders (*see* Chapter 1) should always arouse suspicion of RA. The acromioclavicular, sternoclavicular and manubriosternal joints may all be involved.

The cervical spine
Involvement of the cervical spine with synovitis of the posterior facet joints, neurocentral joints and the atlanto-axial joint results in joint and ligament destruction. This leads to instability of the spine and the risk of subsequent neurological damage to either the spinal cord or nerve roots is high (*Fig.* 5.4). Severe cervical pain often radiates into the shoulders and up into the occiput. This pain may be associated with vertigo and intermittent numbness, paraesthesiae and weakness in the arms and legs, usually precipitated by extension or flexion of the neck, indicating instability in the cervical spine and compression of the spinal cord. Occasionally acute quadriplegia results from cervical dislocation, or fracture of the odontoid peg, weakened by erosive disease (*Fig.* 5.4). This complication requires urgent treatment by external fixation initially with a stiff collar, and then permanent internal fixation surgically. Interestingly, the rest of the spine is rarely involved by rheumatoid arthritis in contradistinction to the seronegative spondarthropathies (*see* Chapter 8).

◀ Cervical spine involvement results in instability and may cause cord compression.

The hip joint
Hip joint involvement, usually symmetrical, can cause considerable disability but is fortunately relatively rare. It presents with bilateral groin pain and tenderness with associated loss of motion of the joints themselves. If marked destructive changes have occurred, deformities, such as flexion and adduction deformities resulting in apparent shortening of the leg, will be seen. It should be noted that a rheumatoid hip tends to 'travel' into the pelvis. This is known as protrusio acetabuli (*Fig.* 5.5), and causes a true shortening of the leg.

◀ Bilateral protrusio acetabuli is a common result of hip joint involvement.

a

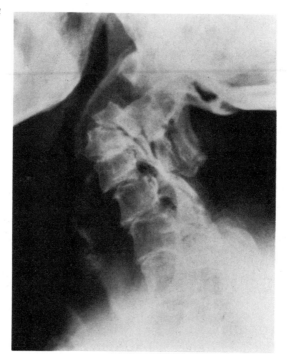

b

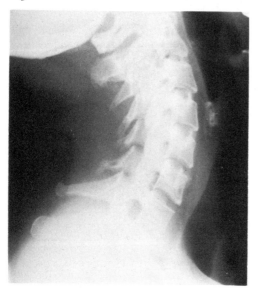 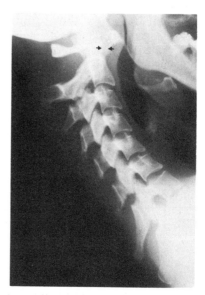

Fig. 5.4. *a*, Gross rheumatoid cervical spine involvement showing subluxation resulting in acute quadriplegia. *b*, Less severe changes showing subluxation of the atlanto-axial articulation on flexion of the neck (arrowed is the gap occurring between the body of the atlas and the odontoid peg. This normally does not exceed 3 mm).

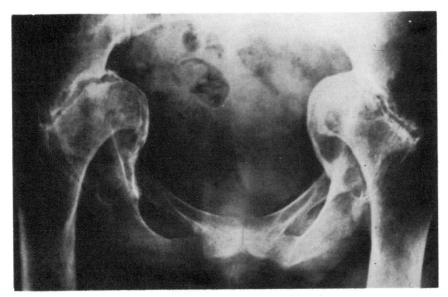

Fig. 5.5. RA involvement of the hips showing loss of 'joint space' and protrusio acetabuli. Note absence of osteophytes.

The knee joint

The knee joint is commonly involved and is a major cause of loss of mobility in the disease. Recurrent attacks of synovitis and resultant cartilage loss cause deformity of the joint. The most common of these is a valgus deformity caused by loss of cartilage and/or bone in the lateral compartment of the knee joint. Varus deformities are also seen (cartilage loss from the medial compartment). Fixed flexion deformities are common. The joints frequently become unstable due to a combination of a ligamentous laxity or destruction, articular cartilage loss and loss of muscle power. Instability can be gross and is one of the major factors to be taken into account when surgical repair is being contemplated.

◀ Instability and pain in the knee joint are major disabling factors in RA.

Popliteal cysts are sometimes seen (developing either as an extension of the knee joint itself or by growth of a semimembranosus bursa) (*see* Chapter 1). They can be enormous, extending well down into the calf (*Fig.* 5.6). Rupture of a popliteal cyst causes *sudden* calf pain with swelling and tenderness that can mimic deep venous thrombosis.

◀ Rupture of a popliteal (Baker's) cyst into the calf can mimic DVT.

The feet and ankle joints

Rheumatoid involvement of the foot is extremely common but patients often overlook pain in their

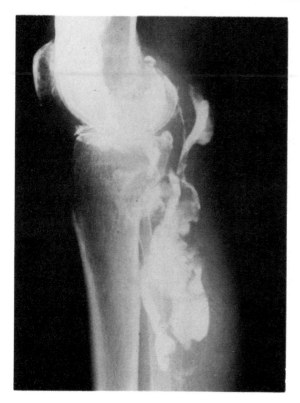

Fig. 5.6. Popliteal cyst extending into the calf in a patient with rheumatoid involvement of the knee. The radiograph was taken after injecting contrast medium into the joint.

feet until quite major deformities and disability have developed. The metatarsophalangeal joints become dislocated and the toes deviate laterally and dorsally, and are flexed at the DIP joints. This is known as 'clawing' (*Fig.* 5.7). As a result of this the patient walks very painfully on the heads of his metatarsals and tender callosities form. The longitudinal arch is also lost, resulting in flat feet. The ankle joint itself is only rarely involved but may become secondarily deformed. The subtalar joint, however, is often involved and valgus deformity secondary to a valgus deformity of the ipsilateral knee is common.

Extra-articular manifestations
These are numerous, important and can be life-

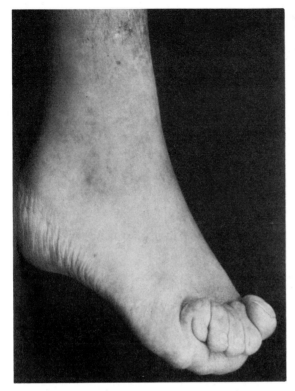

Fig. 5.7. Severe RA changes in the feet.

threatening. Although primarily a disease of synovial membranes, rheumatoid arthritis often develops
as a systemic disease and for this reason the term
rheumatoid disease is to be preferred to 'arthritis'.
Many of the extra-articular manifestations can be
explained on the basis of a vasculitis stimulated by
immune-complex deposition in small blood vessels.
These immune-complexes can be shown to comprise
rheumatoid factor (*see* Laboratory Investigations),
other immunoglobulins and complement. They are
very variable in concentration but can be detected in
the blood of most patients with active rheumatoid
disease. A brief outline of the major extra-articular
manifestations now follows.

Skin manifestations
Subcutaneous *rheumatoid nodules* are found over
any bony prominence that is subject to external
pressure and they are one of the commonest
extra-articular manifestations of the disease. The

◀ Subcutaneous rheuma-
toid nodules occur over any
bony 'pressure' point.

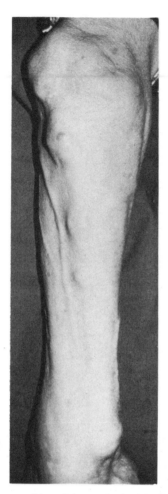

Fig. 5.8. Rheumatoid nodules over the olecranon — the classic site, but they can occur over any bony prominence.

classic site for them is over the olecranon (*Fig.* 5.8) but they are also seen over the occiput, scapulae, Achilles tendons and in flexor tendons of the fingers where they cause 'triggering'. Triggering occurs when the fingers are flexed and the nodule associated with the tendon becomes trapped within the flexor sheath but is suddenly released, like a trigger, on extension. Nodules are sometimes attached to the periosteum of nearby bone and then become relatively fixed. Histologically they comprise a central area of necrosis which contains immunoglobulins (including rheumatoid factor), fibrin and fragmented collagen fibres, surrounded by a palisade of giant cells, interspersed with lympho-cytes and plasma cells, and by fibrous tissue.

Vasculitic lesions are manifested in the skin as small digital infarcts most commonly seen in the nail folds and pulps of the fingers (*Fig.* 5.9), or larger areas of skin necrosis and ulceration, particularly around the ankle (*Fig.* 5.10). Occasionally massive lower limb ulceration occurs which can be life-threatening.

Ocular manifestations

Keratoconjunctivitis sicca (dry eyes) is the most common ocular manifestation and is seen in at least 15% of cases. It is a result of diminished tear secretion which can be detected by a simple bedside test designed by Schirmer (*Fig.* 5.11). In this test a strip of sterile filter paper of standard pore size is placed over the lower lid and the patient asked to close his eyes gently. After 5 minutes the paper is removed and the length of the wetted area is measured. If this is less than 5 mm diminished tear secretion is present, less than 10 mm should be regarded with suspicion. Diminished tear secretion often results in secondary corneal abrasions which can go onto blindness unless treated effectively with

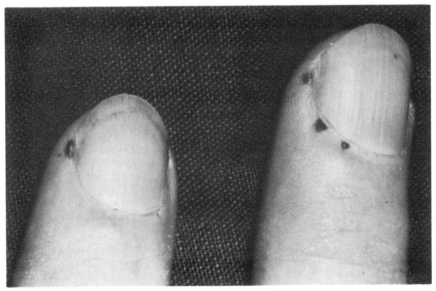

Fig. 5.9. Nail fold infarcts in a patient with rheumatoid vasculitis.

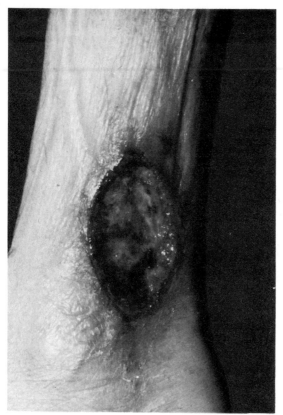

Fig. 5.10. A vasculitic ulcer above the ankle in a patient with severe deforming seropositive rheumatoid disease.

methyl cellulose eye drops ('artificial tears'). When keratoconjunctivitis sicca is associated with diminished salivary secretion and dryness of the mouth (*xerostomia*) in a patient with rheumatoid arthritis it is known as *Sjögren's syndrome*. Inflammation of the sclera (*scleritis*) is an important and sometimes painful ocular manifestation of rheumatoid arthritis. Recurrent attacks of scleritis were thought to lead to a thinning of the sclera (*scleromalacia*) (*Fig.* 5.12) and this is seen as patches of blueness in the sclera as the pigment of the choroid becomes visible. Other explanations such as alteration in the structure of the ground substance of the sclera resulting in increased lucency are probably more accurate. Scleritis must be promptly recognized and treated with steroid eye drops. Nodules may also occur in the sclera and are often associated with scleritis (*nodular scleritis*) and

◄ Sjögren's syndrome may result in irreversible corneal scarring unless promptly treated with artificial tears.

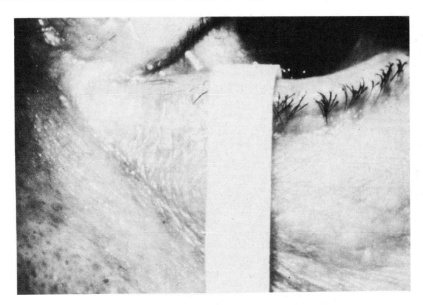

Fig. 5.11. Schirmer's test for diminished tear secretion.

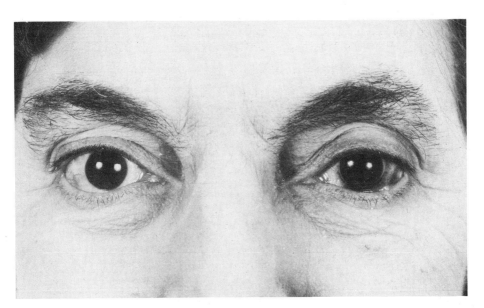

Fig. 5.12. Photograph of the eyes of a rheumatoid patient with scleromalacia (right) and scleritis (left).

it is these lesions that may result in perforation of the globe (*scleromalacia perforans*). *Episcleritis* is inflammation within the superficial layers of the sclera. It tends to be painless but is usually associated with conjunctival injection as a secondary effect. It is not as damaging as scleritis which is a full-thickness inflammation. Uveitis is very rare in RA as compared with its prevalence in seronegative arthritis (*see* Chapter 7). Retinitis is also rare.

◀ Uveitis is rare in RA in contrast to its prevalence in seronegative spondarthritis.

Cardiac manifestations

Pericardium
A *pericarditis* is not uncommon in RA, and one post-mortem survey revealed an incidence as high as 20%. Clinically significant pericardial disease is, however, rare. Pericardial pain, associated with a pericardial rub, may last some months but usually settles spontaneously. Occasionally cardiac tamponade, occurring suddenly as a result of a pericardial effusion and requiring urgent drainage, is seen. *Constrictive pericarditis* is a rare sequela and isolated rheumatoid nodules may occur in the pericardium.

◀ Pericarditis is the commonest cardiac complication of RA.

Myocardium
Inflammation of the myocardium with nodule formation can cause *conduction defects* and an acute *myocarditis* may occur. Both complications are rare.

Endocardium
Rheumatoid (as opposed to rheumatic) *endocarditis* is rare. It usually involves the aortic valve giving rise to lone aortic incompetence but the mitral valve may also be affected and rheumatoid nodule formation in the valve cusps and endocardium can give rise to thrombo-embolism. Rheumatoid nodules may also form the focus of subacute bacterial endocarditis.

◀ Rheumatoid endocarditis may cause valvular damage and predispose to subacute bacterial endocarditis.

Pulmonary manifestations

Pleura
Pleural effusions are not uncommon in RA and can be accompanied by a clinical pleurisy. They can antedate the onset of the arthritis and their true nature will be missed unless the fluid is analysed for

◀ Pleural effusions are common in RA (up to 20%). They are positive for rheumatoid factor and have a high cell count.

rheumatoid factor. The sugar content of the fluid is low, and a polymorpholeucocytosis can cause confusion with infective pleurisy, but the fluid is sterile on culture. Nodules may occur in the pleura.

Lung parenchyma

Fibrosing alveolitis which may lead to a diffuse interstitial fibrosis and 'honeycomb lung' does occur in RA, usually in patients with severe seropositive disease. Patients present with increasing dyspnoea and have characteristic end-inspiratory crepitations on deep inspiration. Rarely patients die in respiratory failure. An *acute bronchiolitis* occurs and carries a poor prognosis, but is fortunately very rare.

Rheumatoid nodules can form in lung tissue and can be multiple and large, simulating the cannon-ball secondaries of carcinoma on radiography. They can also undergo necrosis and cavitation when they have the appearance of a TB focus. When they occur in a patient with dust disease, usually a coal miner with pneumoconiosis, it is known as *Caplan's syndrome*.

◄ Rheumatoid nodules in the lung parenchymas can mimic secondary deposits and cavitating tuberculosis foci.

Neurological manifestations

The patient with rheumatoid disease can present neurologically in several ways (*Table* 5.1). The most common presentation is a *carpal tunnel syndrome* and in some cases this is the initial symptom of the disease. It is caused by compression of the median nerve (entrapment neuropathy) under the flexor retinaculum at the wrist by inflammatory rheumatoid synovial tissue. A similar entrapment neuropathy occurs at the ankle when the posterior tibial

Table 5.1. Neurological manifestations of rheumatoid disease

1. Entrapment neuropathies, e.g. carpal and tarsal tunnel syndromes
2. Mild distal sensory neuropathy
3. Severe sensorimotor neuropathy (mononeuritis multiplex)
4. Upper motor neurone lesions due to spinal cord compression in the cervical spine
5. Lower motor lesions due to nerve root compression in the cervical spine

nerve becomes compressed in the tarsal tunnel below the medial malleolus — *tarsal tunnel syndrome* (*see* Chapter 1). The next most common is a *mild distal sensory neuropathy* presenting as numbness and paraesthesiae, usually in the feet. The incidence of the neuropathy when diligently sought clinically is much higher than its symptomatology would suggest. A *severe sensorimotor neuropathy* involving large nerves is much less common but much more dramatic in its presentation. The patient is usually male and often suffers sudden foot drop due to the involvement of the common peroneal nerve. Other nerves may also be affected, e.g. radial and ulnar, and the condition can then be regarded as a *mononeuritis multiplex*. Both these forms of neuropathy are thought to be caused by the deposition of immune complexes in the vasa nervorum resulting in thrombosis. Histological evidence for this aetiology is, however, not strong and other pathological processes probably operate.

Quadriplegia, resulting from compression of the spinal cord after atlanto-axial dislocation, is an equally dramatic presentation. The spinal cord may also be compressed at other levels in the neck due to severe instability caused by rheumatoid involvement of the posterior facet joints and ligamentous and bone destruction. In most cases, there is a previous history of transient weakness or paraesthesia in the arms and legs, and it is imperative to perform full neurological examination and take flexion and extension views of the cervical spine in order that such cases can be detected before irreversible neurological damage occurs (*see* Clinical section on established disease).

◄ Serious cervical cord compression is heralded by transient paraesthesiae and weakness in the arms and legs – treatment at this stage with a cervical collar can help prevent the disastrous complication of quadriplegia.

Reticulo-endothelial manifestations (*Table* 5.2)
The most common manifestation is a *normochromic, normocytic anaemia* which mirrors the severity and the chronicity of the disease. There is defective utilization of iron in rheumatoid arthritis. Iron appears to be trapped in the reticulo-endothelial system and is unavailable for haemopoeisis. Iron stores in the bone marrow are usually normal or increased and serum iron tends to be low while iron-binding capacity is normal. Under these circumstances administration of iron preparations is futile

◄ Normochromic, normocytic anaemia is the most common. It is unresponsive to iron therapy which can result in serious iron overload.

Table 5.2. Reticulo-endothelial complications of rheumatoid disease

1. Anaemia
   a. Normochromic, normocytic (of chronic disease)
   b. Iron deficiency
      i. Secondary to defective utilization of iron
      ii. Secondary to gastrointestinal blood loss
   c. Coombs' positive haemolytic anaemia
2. Lymphadenopathy
3. Splenomegaly
4. Splenomegaly and neutropenia — Felty's syndrome

and can give rise to serious iron overload. A true *iron-deficiency anaemia* (hypochromic, microcytic) may also be present and is almost always due to gastrointestinal blood loss resulting from ingestion of irritating drugs, particularly non-steroidal anti-inflammatory drugs. An anaemia as a result of dietary deficiency is also seen. A Coombs'-positive *haemolytic anaemia* can occur acutely.

◀ A true iron-deficiency anaemia may result from G.I. blood loss secondary to NSAID ingestion.

Lymphadenopathy of regional lymph nodes draining an affected joint(s) is extremely common in rheumatoid disease and histology reveals reactive cellular hyperplasia within the lymph node but no evidence of lymphomatous change. Isolated splenomegaly also occurs but when seen in conjunction with a neutropenia is known as *Felty's syndrome.*

◀ Felty's syndrome:
● rheumatoid arthritis
● splenomegaly
● neutropenia

Renal manifestations
Renal involvement in RA is surprisingly uncommon when one considers the high levels of circulating immune complexes that are sometimes seen in the disease. A rheumatoid glomerulitis is recognized but is very rare. Proteinuria occurring in a patient with RA is most likely due to intercurrent renal tract infection or due to drug toxicity (especially gold or penicillamine but occasionally *analgesic nephropathy* can occur — *see* Treatment). Another cause of proteinuria is *amyloid* deposition of the kidneys. This usually carries a poor prognosis but subclinical amyloid is probably common in rheumatoid disease and can be detected by either a renal or rectal biopsy. Rheumatoid arthritis is the commonest cause of amyloidosis in the western world.

◀ RA is the commonest cause of amyloidosis in the western world.

Laboratory investigations

1. ESR
This is nearly always elevated in acute phases of the disease, and may be the only laboratory abnormality at the onset of the disease.

2. Full blood count
A normochromic, normocytic anaemia is usually seen in established disease and is accompanied by a low serum iron but normal iron-binding capacity. An iron-deficiency picture may develop in addition to this (*see above*).

3. Rheumatoid factor
This is an immunoglobulin, usually of the IgM subclass (though rheumatoid factors in the IgG and IgA subclass have also been identified), which is a true auto-antibody being directed against other immunoglobulin molecules which have somehow undergone a conformational change, i.e. it is an 'antiglobulin'. It is detected in the serum by the Rose–Waaler (sheep-cell agglutination) test (SCAT). Briefly, the basis of this test is illustrated in *Fig.* 5.13. There are several variations of this test, e.g. latex test, in which latex beads are used instead

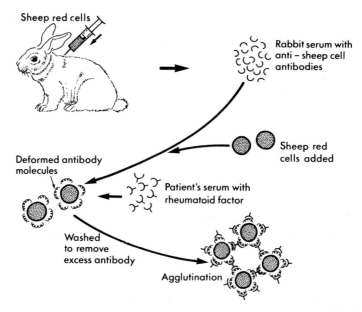

Sheep red cells

Rabbit serum with anti – sheep cell antibodies

Sheep red cells added

Deformed antibody molecules

Patient's serum with rheumatoid factor

Washed to remove excess antibody

Agglutination

Fig. 5.13. Diagrammatic representation of the sheep-cell agglutination test.

of sheep red cells. In the sheep-cell agglutination test the patient's serum is first adsorbed with sheep cells to remove any non-specific (i.e. heterophile) sheep-cell agglutinating antibodies that may be present. In the Differential Agglutination Test (DAT) this problem of heterophile sheep-cell agglutinating antibodies is solved by using sensitized (IgG coated) and non-sensitized cells, the result being expressed as a titre, e.g. 1:64 sensitized, 1:4 unsensitized, result = 1:16. The results of the SCAT are also recorded as titres. A titre of 1:32 or below is usually regarded as negative. Of the normal population 6% will possess rheumatoid factor at these low titres and the incidence increases in the elderly.

◄ The incidence of rheumatoid factor in the normal population increases with age.

Rheumatoid factors are found in 90% of patients at some stage of the disease and these patients are regarded as 'seropositive'. Rheumatoid factors, however, may be undetectable in the early stages and approximately 10% of patients remain 'sero-negative'. They are also found in other disease states (*see Table* 5.3).

◄ Rheumatoid factors are found in 90% of patients but may be absent in the initial stages of the disease.

4. Immunoglobulins

There is usually a rise in immunoglobulins of all subclasses, i.e. *polyclonal rise*.

5. Complement

Serum complement levels are usually normal despite high rates of complement consumption within active rheumatoid joints. Synovial fluid complement levels are usually low. In extensive vasculitis *serum* complement levels may be reduced.

Table 5.3. Other diseases in which rheumatoid factor may be detected

1. SLE
2. Scleroderma
3. Chronic active hepatitis
4. SBE ⎫
5. Leprosy ⎬ chronic infections
6. Pulmonary TB ⎭
7. Syphilis
8. Sarcoidosis
9. Multiple myeloma and other paraproteinaemias
10. Keratoconjunctivitis sicca

6. Synovial fluid analysis (*see* Section on pathology)
- Low viscosity
- High cell count (mainly neutrophils)
- Low glucose
- High protein
- Positive rheumatoid factor

Radiology

Early in the disease, radiographs are frequently normal but it is important to have early radiographs of the *hands* and *feet* to assess future progress of the disease. The earliest joint changes are periarticular soft-tissue swelling and osteoporosis with narrowing of the radiological joint space, indicating cartilage loss. In the next stage subchondral bony erosions occur at the lateral margins of the joint where the synovium is in close contact with the articular surfaces. Finally, gross bony destruction and re-modelling occur and joints, particularly small joints of the hands and feet, become dislocated (*Fig.* 5.14).

◄ Radiographs are frequently normal in the initial stages.

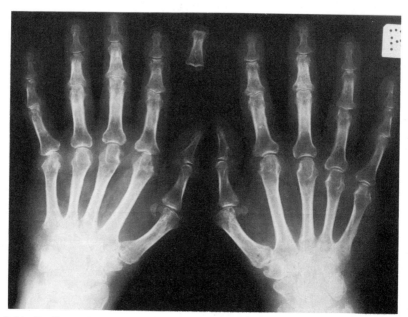

Fig. 5.14. Radiograph of the hands of a patient with rheumatoid arthritis. Note involvement of the MCP and wrist joints with bony erosion, loss of joint space and juxta-articular osteoporosis.

Course and prognosis
The majority of patients follow a chronic course with relapses and remissions in their joint symptoms. Ultimately 50% of patients have little or no deformity and it is worth stressing this to patients once a firm diagnosis of RA has been made; 40% have some residual disability but in only 10% is there severe disability.

Treatment
This is complex and only broad outlines can be given here. Treatment of rheumatoid disease can be divided into five main areas as follows.

Relief of pain
This should be the first aim and is usually the most pressing initial demand by the patient. *Rest* is still very important in the acute exacerbations of the disease. This should be supplemented by drugs, usually analgesics and/or non-steroidal anti-inflammatory drugs. The main emphasis must be in keeping any drug regime as simple as possible. *Paracetamol* 1 g p.r.n. is the least toxic analgesic but *mefenamic acid* may also be used. There are many non-steroidal *anti-inflamatory agents* now available. *Aspirin* has a time-honoured place as an analgesic/anti-inflammatory agent in RA and is indeed very effective providing patients can tolerate the large doses required for maximum benefit (up to 6 g daily). It can be given in a variety of forms but enteric-coated tablets are probably the best. *Indomethacin* is very effective in relief of joint pain and stiffness, particularly early morning stiffness, but suffers a high incidence of gastrointestinal intolerance. It can be given in suppository form which sometimes obviates this intolerance. *Naproxen*, one of the first proprionic acid derivatives to be developed, is an effective and well-tolerated anti-inflammatory drug. There are at least twenty other non-steroidal anti-inflammatory agents available; some in more common usage are ketoprofen, ibuprofen, diclofenac, fenclofenac (which may also have a disease-suppressing effect, *see below*) azopropazone, piroxicam and fenbuffen. All may cause gastrointestinal upset and, less commonly, skin rashes.

◄ Rest in the acute stages is still very important.

Corticosteroids are extremely effective anti-inflammatory agents, but their use in RA should be restricted to the more elderly patients and for especially severe and prolonged episodes in young persons when the disease threatens to disrupt their daily life and capacity to support themselves or their family. The dose should be as low as possible, e.g. prednisolone 7·5 mg or less, and given in an enteric-coated form. The elderly patient can often be adequately maintained on 5 mg on alternate days. In the young patient, steroids should only be prescribed on the understanding that they will be withdrawn as soon as the disease remits or a disease-suppressing agent (*see below*), introduced simultaneously, becomes effective. Intra-articular injections of long-acting corticosteroid preparations such as methylprednisolone acetate and triamcinolone acetonide are particularly useful if single joints are troublesome.

Disease-suppressing or 'long-term agents'

These are drugs which are thought to have a fundamental disease-modifying effect. They are called 'long-term' agents because they take at least 6 weeks to 3 months to have any action on the disease. They are used in patients who have failed to go into a natural remission and who suffer repeated prolonged attacks with evidence of joint destruction.

◀ Disease-suppressing agents (gold, penicillamine) are used in patients with persistently active disease.

Gold was the first drug to be used in this way. It is given by weekly intramuscular injections of the gold salt *sodium aurothiomaleate* at a dose of 50 mg up to a total dose of 1 g. Then it is given fortnightly. A test dose of 10 mg should always be given prior to treatment to ensure that the patient is not allergic to gold. The major side-effects are proteinuria, due to glomerular damage, bone marrow depression, rashes and mouth ulcers (*Table* 5.4). It is mandatory to check for proteinuria before each injection and to perform a full blood count (including a platelet count) fortnightly. The first sign of marrow depression is a fall in the platelet count. Trials are now in progress of an oral preparation of gold.

Penicillamine is an amino acid analogue of cysteine and valine and is distantly related to penicillin. It is capable of dissociating macromolecular complexes and chelating heavy metals. It was first used in Wilson's disease and subsequently in

Table 5.4.   Side-effects of gold and penicillamine therapy

Gold and penicillamine
   Rashes
   Mouth ulcers
   Proteinuria
   Bone marrow suppression
      (thrombocytopaenia neutropenia)

Penicillamine (common)
   Loss of taste
   Gastrointestinal intolerance
      (nausea and vomiting)

Penicillamine (rare)
   Myasthenia gravis
   Drug-induced SLE
   Pneumonitis

cystinuria. It was not used in rheumatoid arthritis until 1965. Its action is thought to be similar to that of gold and it has a latent period of at least 3 months before any effect on the disease can be seen. It is given initially in a dose of 125 mg daily increasing gradually to 750 mg or 1 g if necessary. Because of its slow action, dosage should not be adjusted more frequently than monthly. Most patients can be maintained on a dose of between 125 mg and 500 mg. Its spectrum of side-effects is similar to that of gold with the addition of gastrointestinal intolerance and some other rarer side-effects listed in *Table* 5.4. Patients often complain of a loss or change in taste on starting treatment, but this usually recovers after a few weeks. Fortnightly blood tests and weekly urine tests are mandatory just as with gold treatment and patients should be closely supervised throughout their treatment.

Hydroxychloroquine, initially developed as an antimalarial, is also an effective long-term agent in RA. Its mode of action is unknown. The dose is 200 mg b.d. for 6 months, reducing to 200 mg daily thereafter. The main side-effects are deposition in the cornea leading to opacification and rarely a retinopathy which can lead to blindness. Both these side-effects are dose related and as the drug is cumulative the total daily maintenance dose should not exceed 400 mg and 6-monthly eye checks should be made. The corneal deposition regresses when the drug is stopped. Other side-effects include skin rashes, occasionally exfoliative dermatitis (it there-fore should *not* be given to patients with psoriasis), gastrointestinal intolerance, tinnitus, vertigo, and rarely amyopathy.

Immunosuppressive agents

Immunosuppressive agents, chlorambucil, cyclo-phosphamide and azathioprine, have all been used in aggressive rheumatoid disease. Their place in the treatment of rheumatoid disease is still widely discussed but they are at present reserved for the more severe complications, such as life-threatening systemic vasculitis and occasionally for irrepressible deforming joint disease. They are often used in conjunction with corticosteroids and sometimes enable the dose of corticosteroids to be reduced and are in this respect known as *steroid-sparing agents*. Intravenous cyclophosphamide has been used suc-cessfully in healing severe cutaneous vasculitic ulcers.

◄ Immunosuppressive drugs are reserved for more severe irrepressible diseases.

Surgical intervention

The surgeon has a great deal to offer the rheumatoid patient. The major areas in which he can help are the hands, the feet, the knees, the hips and the cervical spine. Hand operations, such as metacarpo-phalangeal joint arthroplasty, wrist fusions and tendon grafts are usually performed to improve function and/or relieve pain. *Knee* and *hip arthro-plasty* are very successful in pain relief and in the majority of cases function is improved as well. *Arthrodesis* of a severely destroyed knee has to be performed in some cases and the results are often very good, usually to the surprise of the patient! Cervical spine operations, e.g. decompressing laminectomy, should be considered in that group of patients with signs of increasing spinal cord com-pression (*see* Clinical section).

◄ The major aims of joint surgery in RA are to pre-vent pain and improve function.

Surgical removal of the diseased synovium — *synovectomy* is sometimes performed as a prophyl-actic measure in the hope of preventing further joint damage. It is usually used in the knees but also in other joints such as the wrists and in the tendon sheaths of the hand. The great drawback of this attractive procedure is that it is impossible to remove all the synovium from a given site and the regrowth of diseased synovium is almost invariable. Nevertheless, it can often provide a means of temporarily halting joint damage. A similar result can be obtained by injecting radioactive substances such as *yttrium 90* into a joint (*radiosynovectomy*).

Supportive physical measures

Physiotherapy is an important adjunct to drug therapy. During an acute exacerbation *rest* still has a vital role to play and passive movements of limbs prevent joint contractures forming. Heat or ice applied to inflamed joints can be extremely soothing. When the acute phase has settled, the aim should be to strengthen muscles acting at the affected joints to minimize any inherent instability.

◄ Physiotherapy is vital to help prevent joint contractures and instability.

Occupational therapy is extremely important in ensuring that a patient maintains as much functional output as possible. The therapist has the vital task of assessing how particular patients will cope in their home or work situation, and how best they can be helped using various aids and appliances. Surgical footwear, cervical collars and supportive splints for unstable and painful joints, all have a place in the long-term management of rheumatoid deformities.

◄ Occupational therapy allows functional assessment of the patient and ensures that maximum benefit is gained from aids and appliances that may be necessary for him/her to return successfully to their home/work environment.

Further Reading

Extra-articular manifestations of rheumatoid arthritis. In: *Clinics in Rheumatic Disease*, Vol. 3, No. 3, December 1977. London, Saunders.

Williams R.C. (1974) Rheumatoid arthritis as a systemic disease. In: *Major Problems in Internal Medicine*, Vol. 4. London, Saunders.

Other connective-tissue diseases

6

Strictly speaking, any disease resulting in damage to connective tissues could be included under this rather nebulous title e.g. rheumatoid arthritis. The term is normally reserved for a group of inflammatory diseases affecting primarily blood vessels, synovial tissue, skin and muscles. They are:
1. Systemic lupus erythematosus
2. Scleroderma (systemic sclerosis)
3. Dermatomyositis
4. Polyarteritis nodosa
5. Mixed connective-tissue disease

Systemic lupus erythematosus (SLE)
This is a systemic disease of unknown aetiology with a female to male ratio of 9:1, which can affect virtually any system in the body. It is characterized by the presence in the serum of antibodies directed against nuclear constituents (antinuclear factors, ANF) and can result in considerable morbidity and mortality.

Pathology
No single pathological lesion is diagnostic of SLE. The basic cause of the tissue damage seen in the disease is thought to be a diffuse vasculitis precipitated by the deposition of immune complexes affecting the small arteries, arterioles and capillaries. This results in thrombosis and tissue necrosis with scarring. The presence of a substance known as *fibrinoid* is often seen in the affected tissue. This comprises fibrin, gammaglobulin and complement

76

proteins and is particularly common in blood vessels. The other notable histological feature of the disease is the *haematoxylin body* which is a product of the in vivo action of the antinuclear factors on tissue cells. This action causes nuclear damage and the nuclear debris so produced is taken up by phagocytic cells and stains characteristically with haematoxylin and eosin. These cells may be seen in peripheral blood films or tissue sections from patients with SLE. This is also the basis of the now outdated in vitro test for the disease, the 'LE cell test'. In this test, normal peripheral blood neutrophils ingest nuclear debris which has become coated with antinuclear factor in a sample of defibrinated blood from a patient with SLE.

Antinuclear factors
Several of these antibodies have now been characterized and although not unique to SLE they are found in 98–99% of SLE patients. They are not species specific and the basic test (*Fig.* 6.1) to detect them uses thin tissue slices of either rat liver or rabbit kidney as substrate (*see Fig.* 6.5). These sections are flooded with test serum. Any antinuclear antibodies present are taken up by the corresponding antigen in the nuclei of the sections. Excess serum is washed off and then the section is flooded with prepared goat antisera containing anti-human IgG labelled with a fluorescein tag. This antibody will react with any human immunoglobulin present in the test system and in a positive test will identify any antinuclear factor which has reacted with the cell nuclei. The section is then viewed under ultraviolet light and the presence of tagged anti-human IgG, signifying a positive test, will be seen as an area of bright green fluorescence. While this test is not specific for SLE, it is very sensitive and is therefore used as a screening test and has now superseded the more specific but less sensitive LE cell test (*see above*). Antinuclear factors are also found in rheumatoid arthritis (20–40%) and other disease states (*see Table* 6.1). The particular antinuclear factor that is pathognomonic of SLE is directed against various purine and pyrimidine base sequences in *double-stranded DNA* and is in the IgG subclass of immunoglobulins. A radio-immune assay

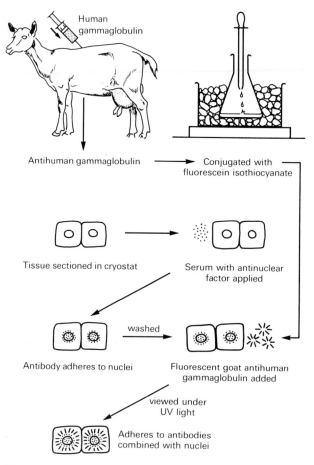

Human gammaglobulin

Antihuman gammaglobulin ⟶ Conjugated with fluorescein isothiocyanate

Tissue sectioned in cryostat

Serum with antinuclear factor applied

washed

Antibody adheres to nuclei

Fluorescent goat antihuman gammaglobulin added

viewed under UV light

Adheres to antibodies combined with nuclei

Fig. 6.1. Immunofluorescent test for antinuclear factors, *see* text for full explanation (*after* Asherson G. L.).

Table 6.1. Other diseases in which antinuclear factors are found

1. Rheumatoid arthritis
2. Keratoconjunctivitis sicca and Sjögren's syndrome
3. Juvenile chronic arthritis
4. Hashimoto's disease
5. Disseminated malignancy
6. Chronic active hepatitis
7. 'Idiopathic' fibrosing alveolitis
8. Myasthenia gravis
9. Leukaemia

is used to detect this specific antibody in the serum by its abilities to bind to double-stranded DNA obtained from bacteria extracts (DNA-binding assay).

◄ Antinuclear factors are a series of antibodies directed against various nuclear antigens. In SLE anti-DNA antibodies are characteristic and detected by a radio-immune assay — DNA-binding assay.

Clinical manifestations

The clinical manifestations are protean and only the more common ones are discussed here.

Constitutional symptoms such as fever, weight loss, tiredness, anorexia and generalized weakness are non-specific but common features.

Musculoskeletal

Of patients with SLE, 95% have musculoskeletal symptoms referable to the musculoskeletal system at some time in the course of the disease and they are common presenting features. A symmetrical arthritis affecting the small joints, sometimes indistinguishable from rheumatoid arthritis, may be the first symptom of active SLE. Arthralgia can be very severe without clinical evidence of synovitis. Tenosynovitis either of the flexor tendons of the fingers or of the extensor tendons of the wrist is sometimes seen. Chronic arthritis can lead to joint deformity secondary to capsular and tendon fibrosis and contracture, but usually without cartilage erosion. This rare deforming arthritis is identical to that described in post-rheumatic fever patients by Jaccoud, and SLE is now the commonest cause of *Jaccoud's arthritis* in the UK. The deformities are similar to those seen in rheumatoid disease but are passively correctable.

A true *myositis* occurs in about 5% of cases and presents as muscle weakness, tenderness and wasting.

◄ 95% of patients have musculoskeletal symptoms.

◄ Arthritis may be indistinguishable from early rheumatoid disease but is non-erosive.

Cardiovascular disease

Raynaud's phenomenon is seen in 25% of patients and may be the presenting feature (*see Fig.* 6.2). True Raynaud's phenomenon occurring in a young woman should always alert one to the possibility of SLE. *Hypertension* secondary to renal involvement is an important cause of morbidity in SLE and

◄ Raynaud's phenomenon occurring for the first time in a young woman may be a presenting feature of SLE.

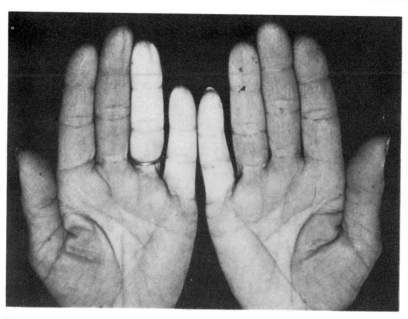

Fig. 6.2. Raynaud's phenomenon. In this patient asymmetrical pallor of the fingers has occurred on cold exposure; symmetrical distribution is more usual.

frequent monitoring of blood pressure and its subsequent control are mandatory in the management of a patient with SLE. Direct cardiac involvement is rare but can take several forms. *Pericarditis*, sometimes with effusion, is the most common but life-threatening cardiac tamponade is rare. Clinically significant *myocarditis* is less common but can result in heart failure. *Verrucous endocarditis* described by Libman–Sacks consists of chronic inflammation in the endocardium which results in fibrosis and damage to the valve cusps, particularly of the mitral valve, leading to mitral regurgitation. The right side of the heart can also be affected and this sometimes helps distinguish SLE endocarditis from rheumatic endocarditis. Subacute bacterial endocarditis may supervene.

Renal involvement

Lupus glomerulonephritis is one of the most serious complications of SLE and accounts for considerable morbidity and mortality, and is still the major cause of death in the disease. Early detection and vigorous treatment can occasionally pay handsome dividends but unfortunately a considerable number of cases

◀ Lupus glomerulo-nephritis carries considerable morbidity and is still the major cause of death. Vigorous treatment is indicated.

follow a relentless downhill course. Histologically the most common lesion is a focal glomerulitis presenting as haematuria on routine urine testing. A membranous glomerulonephritis resulting in proteinuria is also seen with basement membrane deposition of complement and immunoglobulins, including antinuclear factor. Both these types of renal involvement carry a favourable prognosis. Proliferative glomerulonephritis with crescent formation is the least common type and carries a bad prognosis. A nephrotic syndrome can present at any stage and it too carries a bad prognosis, though not invariably so. Renal biopsy is used in assessing prognosis and future management of these patients.

◀ Focal, membranous and proliferative glomerulonephritis may occur, the latter carries the worse prognosis.

Pulmonary involvement

Pleuritic chest pain associated with a pleural rub and later an effusion is the presenting feature in about 50% of patients. A diffuse basal *alveolitis* associated with areas of collapse also occurs and can be rapidly progressive, causing marked reduction of lung volumes ('shrinking lung syndrome'). A further cause of respiratory failure is diaphragmatic involvement resulting in weakness of the diaphragm and marked reduction in vital capacity.

◀ Pleurisy is the most common form of pulmonary involvement.

Skin manifestations (*Table* 6.2)
The cutaneous lesions of SLE usually comprise erythematous macules associated with follicular plugging and later scarring distributed symmetrically over the face, neck and back. The most well-known skin lesion is the erythematous butterfly rash seen on

Table 6.2.   Skin manifestations of SLE

1. Erythematous macules with follicular plugging
2. Photosensitive 'butterfly' rash on cheeks
3. Discoid lupus erythematosus — as in (1) but no systemic involvement
4. Alopecia (especially in active phases of the disease)
5. Livedo reticularis
6. Thrombophlebitis
7. Vasculitis
8. Erythema nodosum
9. Bullous eruptions
10. Buccal ulceration

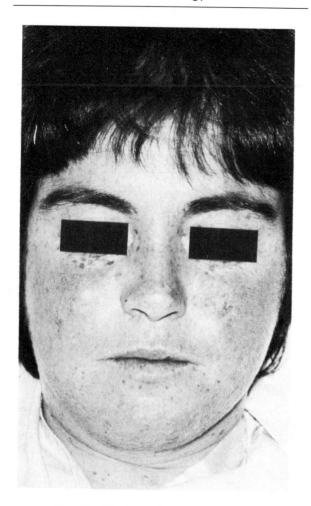

Fig. 6.3. The butterfly rash of SLE.

the face (*Fig.* 6.3) but in its classic form it occurs in less than half the cases. Histologically there is inflammation of the skin capillaries, deposits of immunoglobulins including antinuclear factor and complement at the epidermal–dermal junction which can be readily seen by immunofluorescence staining techniques, both in involved and uninvolved skin (this is known as the *lupus band test*). The condition *discoid lupus erythematosus* (DLE) is related to SLE but the lesions are confined to the skin. Of discoid LE patients 5%, however, develop SLE and over a third can be shown to have Raynaud's phenomenon, arthralgia, raised ESR and

◄ The lupus band test, used diagnostically, detects immunoglobulin deposition at the epidermal–dermal junction.

◄ 5% of patients with discoid LE develop SLE.

positive antinuclear factors. A relative *alopecia* (rarely total) is common, and the comment 'my hair is falling out, doctor' is often spontaneously voiced by young women during the active phases of the disease. Other skin lesions, such as livedo reticularis, together with thrombophlebitis, vasculitis (including erythema nodosum), buccal ulceration and bullous eruptions have all been described but are non-specific.

◄ Relative alopecia is common in active disease.

Neurological manifestations

Symptoms due to central nervous system involvement have become increasingly recognized and cerebral involvement carries a poor prognosis rivalling that of renal disease.

◄ Cerebral involvement carries a poor prognosis.

Psychotic illness, *convulsions* and *cranial nerve lesions* can all occur. Mild *depressive* episodes, sometimes preceding the diagnosis of SLE for many years, are common. A sensorimotor peripheral neuropathy may occur.

Ocular lesions

Keratoconjunctivitis sicca is detectable by an abnormal Schirmer test in about 50% of patients (*see* Chapter 5). A retinitis, best demonstrated by fluorescein angiography, results in exudates (known as cytoid bodies) and haemorrhages, but blindness is very rare.

◄ Positive Schirmer test in 50% of patients.

Reticulo-endothelial system (*Table* 6.3)

The commonest abnormality is a normochromic, normocytic anaemia. A Coombs'-positive haemolytic anaemia also occurs. *Neutropenia*, and more

Table 6.3. Reticulo-endothelial system manifestations of SLE

1. Normochromic, normocytic anaemia
2. Coombs'-positive haemolytic anaemia
3. Neutropenia
4. Lymphopenia
5. Coagulation abnormalities
6. Lymphadenopathy
7. Splenomegaly (15%)

commonly *lymphopenia*, occur in about 50% of patients at some stage of the disease and antibodies directed against neutrophils can sometimes be demonstrated in these patients. *Thrombocytopenia* is less common but may be a presenting feature of the disease. Any of these haematological abnormalities occurring spontaneously in a young female should always raise the suspicion of SLE. Rare *abnormalities of coagulation* caused by the formation of antibodies to various components of the coagulation cascade can occasionally give rise to a clinically significant bleeding disorder, which is usually mild, though when associated with concurrent thrombocytopenia can be severe and difficult to manage. Paradoxically intravascular coagulation also occurs particularly in the pulmonary vessels, though it too is fortunately rare.

Lymphadenopathy is not uncommon, particularly during acute exacerbations of the disease. Biopsy reveals a non-specific lymphadenitis. *Splenomegaly* occurs in about 15% of patients. Histology of the involved spleen provides one of the few absolutely characteristic lesions of the disease, that of concentric peri-arteriolar fibrosis of the arteries in the Malpighian corpuscles — the so-called *onion skin lesions*.

◄ Neutropenia and lymphopenia in 50% of patients.

◄ Clinically relevant clotting disorders are rare but becoming increasingly recognized.

Drug-induced SLE

Patients with SLE commonly show drug hypersensitivity reactions. In addition to this, some drugs are known to precipitate a syndrome closely resembling idiopathic SLE which is usually much milder and one which fortunately resolves in the majority of cases after withdrawal of the offending drug. The number of drugs known to do this is ever-increasing; the chief among them are hydralazine, procainamide, methyldopa, isoniazid, penicillamine and some anticonvulsants. These drugs are all capable of inducing the formation of antinuclear factor but it is usually directed against single-stranded DNA not double-stranded DNA as in idiopathic SLE. Many patients taking these drugs develop positive antinuclear factor tests some time during the course of their treatment, particularly those taking hydralazine but only a few will develop symptoms and signs of the disease.

◄ Drug hypersensitivity is common, especially salicylates.

◄ Formation of antibodies to single stranded DNA is characteristic of drug-induced SLE.

Laboratory investigations

Haematological
1. A full blood count may reveal a normochromic, normocytic anaemia in longstanding disease.
2. A mild haemolytic anaemia may also be seen and in these patients the direct Coombs' test will be positive.
3. Neutropenia and/or lymphopenia may be present.
4. Thrombocytopenia.
5. The ESR is often elevated during exacerbations of the disease though in general correlates poorly with disease activity.

Immunological tests
In a patient clinically suspected of having SLE but with a persistently negative antinuclear factor screening test, the diagnosis should be regarded with suspicion. Such patients have been reported but are extremely rare. Where possible, *anti-double-stranded DNA antibodies* should also be sought to confirm the diagnosis (*see* Pathology). *Complement* levels are often low in active disease due to an increased rate of complement consumption and are a useful guide to monitoring disease activity and response to treatment in individual patients. For the same reason, levels of anti-double-stranded DNA antibodies can be monitored. As one would expect, *immunoglobulin levels* are often high in patients with SLE, particularly the IgG subclass. Occasionally, low levels of IgA are found but the significance is not fully understood.

◄ Complement levels may be low in active disease. Hypergammaglobulinaemia is common.

Treatment
In the majority of patients the disease is mild and only requires symptomatic treatment. The arthritis is usually adequately controlled with non-steroidal anti-inflammatory drugs though aspirin and aspirin-containing compounds should be avoided as there is an increased risk of hepatotoxicity. Patients with Raynaud's phenomenon have usually learnt to avoid rapid changes of temperature and to wear mittens when they go out in the cold. Patients with skin involvement should avoid strong sunlight as ultra-violet radiation can exacerbate the rash. The wearing of wide-brimmed hats and the use of barrier creams are usually effective prophylactic measures.

◄ In the majority of patients the disease is mild and only requires symptomatic treatment.

It is only the patients with particularly active disease, or those who develop major complications, that require more aggressive therapy. In the persistently active group, *corticosteroid therapy* is often indicated and low dose regimes (not more than 7·5 mg per day) are usually effective in relieving symptoms. *Hydroxychloroquine* is also effective in this group, particularly in those patients with skin involvement. In the patients with life-threatening complications, such as renal involvement, high dose steroids (e.g. up to 80 mg prednisolone a day) are usually required for short periods to tide the patient over a relapse. Other forms of treatment used in this group are:

◀ Corticosteroids are used only for persistently active disease or life-threatening complications.

- 'pulse' high dose intravenous steroid therapy
- immunosuppressive agents, e.g. azathioprine, cyclophosphamide
- plasmapheresis (plasma exchange).

Infection is common in SLE patients due to their altered and defective immune mechanisms (particularly cell-mediated immunity) and should always be sought in patients who relapse and antibiotic therapy promptly instituted. Sulphonamides and penicillin should be avoided as they can both exacerbate SLE.

◀ SLE patients are more prone to infections due to a defective immune mechanism (particularly depressed cell-mediated immunity).

Scleroderma (progressive systemic sclerosis)
This is a disease principally affecting the skin, though it often progresses to involve other organs such as the gut, heart, lungs and kidneys and in these cases the term 'progressive systemic sclerosis' is used. It is more common in females than males.

Aetiology
The aetiology is unknown but the disease is characterized by inflammation and progressive fibrosis of the subcutaneous connective tissues. It is usually accompanied and often preceded by Raynaud's phenomenon and abnormalities of the skin capillaries. Abnormal collagen biosynthesis and degradation have been described and this is primarily responsible for the increase in the fibrous elements within the connective tissues. The collagen produced by scleroderma patients has a different macromolecular structure from that of normal collagen in that the number of cross-links between the protein molecules making up the collagen fibres is increased, making it much less biodegradable.

Clinical features

Although in the majority of patients the brunt of the disease falls on the skin, it is becoming increasingly recognized that the typical thickened and inelastic skin is a late manifestation and is often preceded, sometimes by many years, by other changes in the subcutaneous connective tissues, such as Raynaud's phenomenon, generalized subcutaneous oedema and telangiectasia. The clinical features of the disease as they affect various organs will now be discussed.

◀ The typical skin changes of scleroderma are a late manifestation of the disease.

Skin

Sclerodermatous skin is thick, inelastic and shiny. The latter feature, in part, is due to the loss of hair follicles and sweat glands as they become involved in the fibrotic process. The skin of the fingers is most commonly involved and leads to tapering (*sclerodactyly*), which is made more prominent by the loss of the pulp of the finger-tip. The inelasticity of the skin makes fine finger movement difficult and can cause considerable disability for the patient. The skin of the face is also often involved and results in puckering around the edges of the mouth and a generally 'pinched' look as the skin over the bridge of the nose and forehead becomes involved (*Fig. 6.4*). Patients sometimes spontaneously complain of being unable to open their mouth fully (*microstomia*), and some have difficulty in chewing. Inelasticity of the lips and cheeks results in poor dental hygiene and incidence of severe dental caries is high. Intubation during general anaesthesia can be a problem. *Telangiectasia*, seen particularly over the fingers and face, is common. Calcium may also become deposited in the subcutaneous tissues and can lead to skin ulceration and secondary infection. The combination of calcinosis, Raynaud's phenomenon, sclerodactyly and telangiectasia is known as the *CRST syndrome*.

◀ A variant of scleroderma, the CRYST syndrome comprises:
● Dermal calcinosis
● Raynaud's phenomenon
● Sclerodactyly
● Telangiectasia

A localized form of scleroderma called *morphoea* usually affects areas of the trunk, and is seen as sheets or lines of thickened inelastic skin. In the majority of these cases there is no systemic involvement and the outlook is very good.

Renal

Arteriolar obliteration, particularly of the interlobular vessels, leads to scarring, severe hyper-

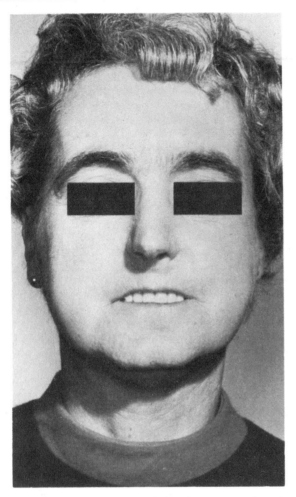

Fig. 6.4. Sclerodermatous facies. Note narrowing of mouth and 'pinched' look around nose.

tension and renal failure. Renal involvement is often rapidly fatal and careful monitoring of blood pressure and renal function is mandatory.

◄ Renal involvement is often rapidly fatal but fortunately rare.

Gastrointestinal
Abnormal oesophageal motility with diminished peristalsis can be demonstrated on barium swallow in 75% of patients. This can cause dysphagia, which occasionally may be severe and result in aspiration of food into the bronchial tree and subsequent pneumonia. *Hiatus hernia* is another common finding on barium examination and acid reflux can often be a troublesome symptom occasionally

◄ 75% of patients have abnormal oesopagheal motilities.

leading to oesophageal stricture requiring dilatation. Duodenal and ileal dilatation with stasis and bacterial overgrowth can lead to malabsorption syndrome. *Keratoconjunctivitis sicca* (*see* Chapter 5) can also occur with xerostomia resulting in further trouble with mastication, swallowing and dental caries.

◀ Bacterial colonization of the upper G. I. tract can lead to malabsorption.

Peripheral vessels
Raynaud's phenomenon is seen in 80% of patients with scleroderma and often antedates the onset of systemic involvement by years. Raynaud's phenomenon is characterized by pallor, followed by cyanosis of the extremities on exposure to the cold. The intense vasoconstriction causing these changes gradually resolves and is followed by a period of vasodilatation when the extremities become suffused, swollen and painful. The temperature changes needed to precipitate an attack can be very minor. Emotional upset can also trigger an attack. The vasoconstriction may be so pronounced and prolonged as to produce areas of infarction in the fingers and toes, though this is rare. Why the peripheral blood vessels should react in this way is unknown but a local vascular wall defect and hypersensitivity to noradrenaline may be a factor. Other causes of Raynaud's phenomenon are shown in *Table* 6.4.

◀ Raynaud's phenomenon which can be a presenting feature occurs in 80% of patients.

◀ Raynaud's phenomenon is common in connective-tissue diseases, particularly scleroderma and also occurs in rheumatoid disease.

Pulmonary
A reduced diffusing capacity is the earliest indication of lung involvement in scleroderma and is a common finding. However, lung involvement severe enough to cause dyspnoea is a late feature. At this stage, *pulmonary fibrosis* can usually be detected on a chest radiograph and in later severe cases changes of honeycombing may be seen. *Pulmonary hypertension* may develop, resulting in cor pulmonale. Pleural involvement is rare.

◀ Abnormalities in pulmonary diffusion are common

◀ Pleural involvement is rare in scleroderma.

Table 6.4. Causes of Raynaud's phenomenon

1. Idiopathic
2. Connective tissue diseases — especially scleroderma
3. Rheumatoid arthritis
4. Cryoglobulinaemia (precipitation of immunoglobulins in peripheral circulation on cold exposure)
5. Vibrating tools

Cardiac
Scleroderma may affect the heart in several ways.
Cor pulmonale results from pulmonary involvement.
Systemic hypertension and hypertension resulting
from renal involvement can cause hypertensive heart
disease. Direct involvement of the heart is well
documented, though its exact frequency is unknown.
Pericarditis, myocarditis and a *cardiomyopathy* all
occur and ECG abnormalities are sometimes seen
early in the disease.

Musculoskeletal
Arthralgia and arthritis are seen in 30% of
scleroderma patients early in the disease. The
arthritis is usually mild and non-destructive. Tendon
sheath involvement with fibrosis can result in
creaking noises in the hands, digital deformities and
trigger finger. *Myositis* is being increasingly recognized as part of the clinical spectrum of scleroderma
but some authorities believe that these patients
belong to another disease group called 'mixed
connective-tissue disease' (*see below*).

◀ 30% of patients have
mild arthritis. Tendon
sheath involvement is
more disabling.

Investigations
Laboratory tests and radiographs provide very little
positive diagnostic help in scleroderma. There may
be a normochromic, normocytic anaemia and the
ESR is elevated in over two-thirds of patients.
Immunoglobulin levels may be increased. The
antinuclear factor test is positive in low titre in
40–60% of patients and when the staining pattern is
examined closely this is usually found to be of a
speckled type rather than the homogeneous type
which is more characteristic of SLE (*Fig. 6.5*).
Anti-DNA antibodies are found in 18% of patients.
Antibodies to ribonuclear protein (RNP), however,
are much more common (*see* section on Mixed
connective-tissue disease). Complement levels are
normal.

◀ ANF is positive in
40–60% of patients. Anti-
DNA antibodies in 18%.
The ANF staining pattern is
characteristically speckled.

Radiology
Radiographs of the hands may reveal soft-tissue
calcification and resorption of the tufts of the
terminal phalanges and associated loss of the soft
tissues. Chest radiography shows a reticular shadow-
ing in the lower zones characteristic of pulmonary
fibrosis in the patients with extensive lung involvement. This may lead to cavitation and honeycombing. Barium examination of the GI tract is described
above in the clinical section.

◀ Hand radiographs may
show soft-tissue calcification and resorption of the
terminal phalanges.

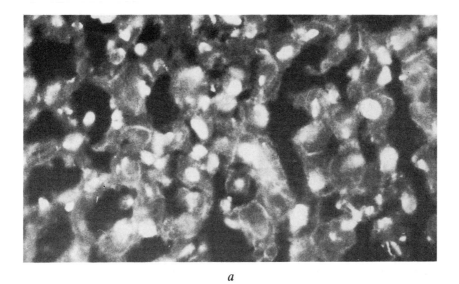

a

b

Fig. 6.5. Immunofluorescent patterns of ANF. *a*, Homogeneous (from a patient with SLE) (substrate, rat kidney, ×60); *b*, Speckled (from a patient with scleroderma) (substrate, rat kidney ×40).

Treatment

This is at present entirely unsatisfactory and purely symptomatic. Nothing halts the disease process, but D-penicillamine (*see* Chapter 5) in high dosages has been claimed to cause regression of some of the fibrosis. Prophylaxis in terms of protecting vulnerable, easily infected skin, and the extremities from the cold are very important measures. Electrically heated mittens are very helpful in the winter months. Increasing the core temperature of the body by wearing a thermal body stocking also gives some protection from Raynaud's phenomenon. Specific vasodilators can be used in severe Raynaud's but they have no long-term effect on the disease process in general. Corticosteroids have a limited use in the disease and are only indicated in those stages where there is acute subcutaneous inflammation with oedema, myositis and possibly pulmonary disease. Standard antacid preparations are used for those patients with oesophageal reflux, and patients with bacterial colonization of the small bowel are given antibiotics, such as neomycin and metronidazole, to sterilize the gut and alleviate malabsorption. *Regular physiotherapy*, much of it self-administered, can help general mobility and prevent more serious contractures, especially of the fingers.

Dermatomyositis and polymyositis

Both these rare diseases are traditionally grouped together as it is likely that they represent a group of diseases with similar clinical features but not necessarily sharing the same aetiology. In both, as their title suggests, there is non-suppurative inflammation in the striated muscle and in dermatomyositis this is associated with a characteristic rash. Both can occur at any age but most commonly between the ages of 30 and 60. Dermatomyositis occurring in adults over the age of 50 may be associated with internal malignancy but this is not so with the childhood form of the disease. Polymyositis alone is seen in conjunction with many other diseases such as scleroderma, SLE, rheumatoid arthritis and viral infections and it is important to rule out these diseases before making a diagnosis of 'idiopathic' polymyositis.

◄ The childhood form of dermatomyositis is not associated with malignancy. It carries a good prognosis.

Aetiology

This is unknown though there is now ample evidence of altered lymphocyte function whereby groups of lymphocytes become 'myotoxic' and have the capability of destroying striated muscle in vitro.

Possible precipitating factors are viral infections, certain drugs and in the case of the skin rash, exposure to sunlight.

Clinical manifestations

Muscle

These vary enormously in their extent and mode of onset. In acute stages there may be considerable systemic upset, fever and weight loss. Proximal muscular weakness is the commonest presenting feature associated with wasting and sometimes tenderness of the limb girdle muscles. The legs tend to be affected before the arms but as the disease progresses other muscle groups, particularly in the spine, become affected. Patients initially find difficulty in getting up from a sitting position and develop a waddling gait. As the weakness begins to affect other muscles even raising the head from the pillow may become difficult. The respiratory muscles can be involved and cause respiratory failure. Bulbar muscle involvement, which is usually a late manifestation, creates difficulty with swallowing and speech. Contractures of the limb muscles develop, particularly in children, and there may be marked muscle atrophy and fibrosis. Examination of the affected muscles always reveals weakness and sometimes tenderness and induration, particularly in those cases with an acute onset. Tendon reflexes are reduced.

◄ Respiratory muscle involvement may cause respiratory failure. Monitoring of FVC is essential

Skin

The skin manifestations of dermatomyositis are also extremely variable. The classic fascial heliotrope (i.e. purple) rash in a butterfly distribution is seen in about 40% of cases. The rash may extend or can be confined to the extensor surfaces of the arms and over the back. The skin becomes thickened and occasionally sclerodermatous and scaling is common often causing diagnostic confusion with eczema. Dermal ulceration may occur and cause scarring. Some patients develop characteristic purple-red, raised, slightly scaly patches over the interphalangeal joints, elbows and knees. These are seen particularly in association with active muscle disease. Nail-fold capillaries are often prominent and telangiectasia seen in the nail folds is not uncommon.

Occasionally the disease can have an explosive onset with swelling of the skin of the face, heliotrope rash and profound muscle weakness and tenderness. The myositis sometimes results in extensive calcification in the interfacial planes of the muscles and in the subcutaneous tissues giving a very characteristic radiological appearance. This feature is particularly common in children.

◀ Calcification of the interfascial planes occurs in myositis, especially in children.

Other clinical features

These include *Raynaud's phenomenon* (in about 30%) and *arthralgia* and/or *arthritis* (in about 30%). When these features are present diagnostic confusion with SLE can result. Pulmonary involvement in the form of a *diffuse alveolitis* carries a poor prognosis.

Investigations

1. Muscle enzymes (creatine phosphokinase, aldolase, SGOT and SGPT).
These are all raised in active myositis. They are good indicators of disease activity as is the urinary creatine level.

◀ A rise of muscle enzymes with characteristic histology on muscle biopsy is diagnostic.

2. Muscle biopsy

Histologically the affected muscles show piecemeal necrosis of muscle fibres with inflammatory cell infiltrates and phagocytosis of necrotic fragments of muscle fibres. Fibrosis and regeneration of muscle fibres are seen in areas of healing.

3. Electromyography

This is a useful non-invasive diagnostic test. Characteristic potentials are detectable both at rest and on activity of the involved muscles.

4. ESR

This is often elevated in acute phases of the disease.

5. Full blood count

A neutrophil leucocytosis is sometimes seen during the acute phases.

6. Immunoglobulins

Hypergammaglobulinaemia is a common finding. *Antinuclear factor*. This is usually negative. Antibodies to DNA are not found.

7. *Search for internal malignancy*
This is imperative in adults and should at least include chest radiography, barium meal, barium enema and in women a full gynaecological examination. Such a search should not be undertaken in children as internal malignancy is not an association in this age group.

Treatment
High dose corticosteroid therapy is used and is effective in acute phases of the disease (60–100 mg prednisolone daily). Some patients require varying doses of steroids to maintain remission. The dosage should be titrated against the level of the muscle enzymes. Bed rest is mandatory in the acute phases of the disease. Physiotherapy and splintage both play an important part in preventing muscle contractures, particularly in children. Immunosuppressive therapy, e.g. methotrexate, azathioprine, cyclophosphamide, are used in those patients who are either only partially or completely unresponsive to corticosteroids.

◀ Dose of steroid titrated against level of muscle enzymes.
◀ Bed rest is vital in acute phases.

Mixed connective-tissue disease (MCTD)
The existence of this disease as a separate entity is still open to considerable debate. It represents a clinical overlap syndrome between SLE, scleroderma, and polymyositis and serves to illustrate the considerable variability in these separate conditions. Some authorities believe it to be a variant of SLE with a uniformly favourable prognosis, lack of renal involvement and a good response to steroids. Patients have a high incidence of:
- Raynaud's phenomenon (84%)
- Arthralgias/arthritis – occasionally erosive (96%)
- Abnormal oesophageal motility (70%)
- Myositis (72%)
- Hypergammaglobulinaemia (80%)

These patients also possess antinuclear factors directed against ribonuclear protein (RNP) and in general have low titres of antibodies to DNA. RNP is a saline extractable constituent of nuclei and is known as an *extractable nuclear antigen (ENA)*. Other such antigens exist such as the non-nucleic acid nuclear protein designated as Sm. Antibodies to Sm are found particularly in SLE but not in patients

◀ Patients with MCTD possess antibodies to nuclear ribonuclear protein but have low titres of anti-DNA antibodies. Their ANF usually has a speckled pattern.

with MCTD. Antibodies to RNP are found in some patients with SLE and these patients tend to have a good prognosis. Antibodies to RNP are common in scleroderma but these patients probably represent the MCTD subgroup who do not develop classic systemic sclerosis. Careful serological analysis is therefore important in order to separate these related conditions as the prognosis of the various groups of patients thus defined varies greatly.

Polyarteritis nodosa (PAN)

This is an inflammatory condition involving medium and small arteries resulting classically in nodular aneurysmal dilatations which occasionally can be palpated in subcutaneous vessels, hence the word 'nodosa'. Much of the pathology seen in the disease results from the compromised blood supply of tissues supplied by involved arteries. Any small or medium-sized artery can be affected, thus the clinical manifestations of the disease are widespread and can involve any organ.

Aetiology

This is unknown. Unlike the other connective-tissue diseases PAN is more common in men. Histology of an affected artery shows transmural inflammation and intraluminal thrombosis with surrounding tissue necrosis. Of patients 25–40% can be shown to possess the hepatitis B antigen (HBAg) normally associated with serum hepatitis and there is evidence that some of these patients have deposition of HBAg – antibody complexes in the affected vessels. The significance of this finding is not known at the present time.

◀ More common in men.

Clinical features

These are legion and polyarteritis like SLE is a great mimic. Histological diagnosis is mandatory. Presentation with general malaise, weight loss and a pyrexia of unknown origin (PUO) is common. *Skin rashes* often give diagnostic clues. These can be purpuric or take the form of necrotic ulcers and areas of infarction (*Fig. 6.6*). *Arthralgia* and muscle pains and tenderness are also seen. *Renal involvement* is a common cause of death and also results in severe hypertension, which is often difficult to control. Cardiac complications include *pericarditis* and *myocardial infarction* secondary to coronary

◀ Presentation as 'PUO' is not uncommon.

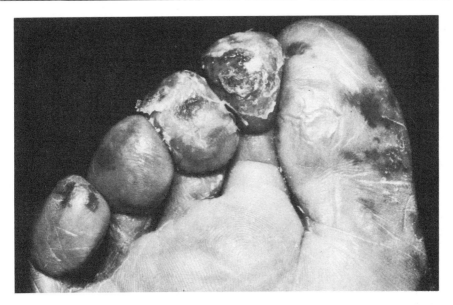

Fig. 6.6. Digital infarction seen in PAN. The patient subsequently died in renal failure.

arteritis. A persistent tachycardia is sometimes present and should always alert one to the possibility of cardiac involvement. The lungs may show transient infiltrates on chest radiography and these patients can present with severe *asthma* or a non-productive cough and chest radiography reports of 'recurrent pneumonia'. The retinal arteries may be affected directly resulting in areas of haemorrhage and exudation. They may also show the ravages of severe hypertension. If the central retinal arteries are affected blindness may result. Patients with PAN may present with an *acute abdomen* and undergo laparotomy before the true basis of their symptoms is realized. Appendicitis, intussusception, gastrointestinal haemorrhage, gastric ulceration, liver infarction, gallbladder infarction, peritonitis and pancreatitis have all been reported and are caused by arteritis affecting various parts of the gastrointestinal tract. A peripheral, mainly motor *neuropathy* is also seen as the result of involvement of the vasa nervorum. Mononeuritis multiplex may also occur (*see* Chapter 5). Cerebral arterial involvement is fortunately rare but can result in hemiplegia, dementia, convulsions, meningitis and cranial nerve palsies. Subarachnoid haemorrhage may also occur.

◀ Persistent tachycardia may indicate cardiac involvement.

◀ May present with an acute abdomen.

◀ PAN may cause a mononeuritis multiplex.

Laboratory investigations

1. ESR
This is usually elevated, sometimes to a very high level.

2. Full blood count
A neutrophilia is common. There may be an absolute eosinophilia, particularly in those patients with pulmonary involvement. Normochromic, normocytic or an iron deficiency anaemia is also seen.

3. Immunoglobulins
Hypergammaglobulinaemia is not uncommon and cryoglobulins may also be detected.

4. Rheumatoid factor
Rheumatoid factor and antinuclear factor are usually negative though an arteritis histologically indistinguishable from PAN may complicate rheumatoid arthritis and SLE.

5. Tissue biopsy
If a diagnosis is to be confirmed, tissue from an affected organ must be obtained and the characteristic histological appearance demonstrated. Muscle biopsy is positive in approximately 40% of patients with tender muscles, but blind muscle biopsy is rarely helpful. Skin, nerve and renal biopsy should be performed if any of these tissues are involved clinically.

6. Coeliac axis angiography
This may demonstrate aneurysms in the smaller arteries of the gut in patients with abdominal symptoms. Renal angiography has also been used in this way in patients suspected of having renal involvement.

7. Urine analysis
Sequential urine analysis is vital as haematuria and proteinuria herald renal involvement and prompt treatment may arrest the progress of the disease before irreversible damage has occurred.

Treatment
Corticosteroids are the only drugs of proven value in this condition. They often have to be used in high dosage. Immunosuppressive drugs such as azathioprine and cyclophosphamide have been used but as yet there is no evidence that they are of benefit in PAN. This is in contradistinction to their use in *Wegener's granulomatosis*. This condition, which has some clinical and pathological features of PAN, is characterized by a generalized arteritis associated with necrosis of the structures of the upper respiratory tract, particularly the nasal mucous membrane and cartilage. Unlike PAN it invariably responds well to immunosuppressive therapy.

◀ Wegener's granulomatosis responds well to immunosuppressive therapy, e.g. cyclophosphamide, azathioprine.

Further Reading
Hughes, G. R. V. (1977) *Connective Tissue Diseases*. Oxford, Blackwell Scientific Publications.

Seronegative arthritides

7

Seronegative arthritides is the name given to a group of arthritides characterized by a consistent absence of rheumatoid factors from the serum (hence seronegative) and a clinical and genetic relationship to ankylosing spondylitis which is now regarded as the central disease of the group. The more exact title of seronegative spondarthritis (implying involvement of the spine as occurs in ankylosing *spondy*litis) helps to distinguish the group from other arthritides which are also seronegative for rheumatoid factor such as gout and osteoarthritis. The diseases in the group are:
1. Ankylosing spondylitis
2. Psoriatic arthritis
3. Enteropathic arthritis (associated with Crohn's disease, ulcerative colitis, Whipple's disease, enteric infections, and intestinal bypass for morbid obesity)
4. Reiter's disease
5. Behçet's syndrome

The inter-relationships of these diseases are illustrated in the Venn diagram (*Fig.* 7.1) — where overlap of the circles implies overlapping symptoms and signs of the various diseases.

Ankylosing spondylitis

This is a disease primarily affecting young males with a male to female ratio of 9:1 and a peak age of onset in teenage. The main brunt of the disease falls on the spine and comprises an inflammation of the sacro-iliac joints (*sacro-iliitis*), posterior facet joints (*spondylitis*), annulus fibrosus of the intervertebral

◀ Onset in teenage. Male: female ratio said to be 9:1 — probably much less than this, e.g. 3:1.

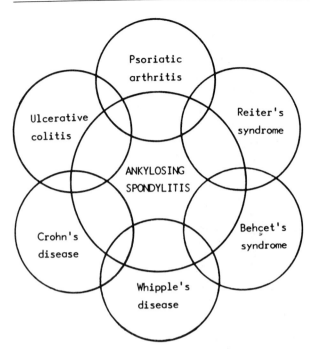

Fig. 7.1. A Venn diagram showing inter-relationship between the seronegative spondarthritides.

discs, and the interspinous ligaments. Extraspinal manifestations of the disease are peripheral arthritis, iritis, aortitis, pulmonary involvement and systemic upset.

Pathology
The basic pathological lesion of ankylosing spondylitis occurs at the *entheses*. These are the sites of attachments of ligaments, tendons and joint capsules to bone. These areas become inflamed and ultimately calcification and new bone formation occur in the soft tissues (an *enthesopathy*). When this calcification occurs in the annulus fibrosus bony bridges are formed between adjacent vertebrae (*syndesmophytes*) and the vertebrae become locked, i.e. ankylosed (*Fig.* 7.2). It is this process of syndesmophyte formation that leads to the rigidity and deformity of the spine seen in patients with ankylosing spondylitis. The process usually starts as an arthritis in the sacro-iliac joints (sacro-iliitis) which become inflamed, sclerotic, eroded and finally

◄ Characteristic new bone formation at the site of entheses.

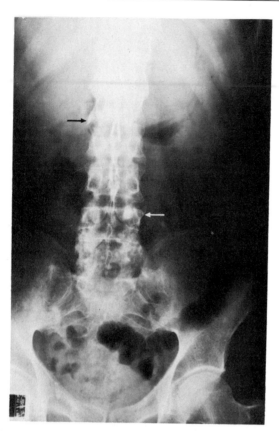

Fig. 7.2. Syndesmophyte formation in the lumbar spine in a patient with ankylosing spondylitis (arrows).

ankylosed. Other areas where enthesopathy occurs are the iliac crests, ischial tuberosities, greater trochanters, patellae and calcanea. A peripheral, large-joint, acute synovitis is not uncommon. Synovial histology is indistinguishable from that of rheumatoid arthritis but pannus formation is not a feature. The synovial fluid is negative for rheumatoid factor.

◀ Peripheral joint synovitis as well as spinal involvement is common.

Aetiology

This is unknown; however, there is clearly a strong genetic influence on the disease. Early family studies pointed to a Mendelian dominant inheritance with approximately 70% penetration of disease manifestations. This is almost certainly an oversimplification of the genetics but a family history of the disease is extremely common. A genetic influence on the disease was further intimated by the discovery that 90–96% of patients with ankylosing spondylitis possess the tissue antigen HLA B27. Human leucocyte-associated (HLA) tissue antigens are carried on virtually all tissue cells but are most readily detected in the laboratory on lymphocytes isolated from the peripheral blood. Seven per cent of the population of this country carry B27 but its prevalence varies from race to race. However, only 1% of B27-positive individuals develop the disease. Thus the possession of B27 alone is insufficient to cause the disease and it is probable that some environmental factor(s) triggers the disease in genetically predisposed individuals. An infective agent, possibly gut borne, seems at present to be the most likely candidate.

◄ Aetiological factors: (*a*), possession of HLA B27 antigen; (*b*), environmental trigger.

Clinical features

Symptoms
Low back pain, often centred over the sacrum and radiating into the groins, buttocks and down the backs of both legs as far as the knees, is the most common presenting symptom. This characteristic pain is caused by *bilateral sacro-iliitis*. The typical patient is a young male who has often had previous episodes of back pain waking him at night and accompanied by spinal stiffness in the morning. These symptoms are sometimes passed off as 'lumbago' but their bilaterality and their exacerbation at *rest* should always alert one to the possibility of ankylosing spondylitis. These features contrast with those of mechanical back pain (*see* Chapter 3) which is usually eased at rest and made worse on exercise. As the disease spreads up the spine pain is experienced at higher levels, particularly around the rib cage which heralds involvement of the costo-vertebral articulations. This pain, which may be an early feature of the disease, is pleuritic in character with bilateral radiation from the thoracic spine around the rib cage, features which help distinguish it from true pleurisy. As chest expansion becomes restricted diaphragmatic excursion increases to compensate and maintain vital capacity. This pheno-menon can be readily observed as the patient's abdomen balloons outwards on each inspiration.

◄ Low back pain and 'stiffness' most comon presenting feature. Worse at rest.

◄ Thoracolumbar involve-ment often presents with bilateral pleuritic type pain.

The cervical spine is usually involved late in the disease and leads to restriction of rotation of the head which can be very disabling. The overall effect of the disease on the spine is to convert it into a rigid piece of bone with loss of the normal curvatures and movement (*Fig.* 7.3). Fortunately total ankylosis is not common and spinal involvement can arrest at any stage.

A peripheral arthritis may occur and precedes the onset of back symptoms in 10–20% of patients. It usually affects the hips and the knees and can occur as an *acute monoarthritis*. Thus in any young male presenting with a non-infective seronegative mono-arthritis a diagnosis of ankylosing spondylitis must

◀ Peripheral large joint arthritis may precede back symptoms.

◀ Always suspect diagnosis in young male with mono-articular synovitis.

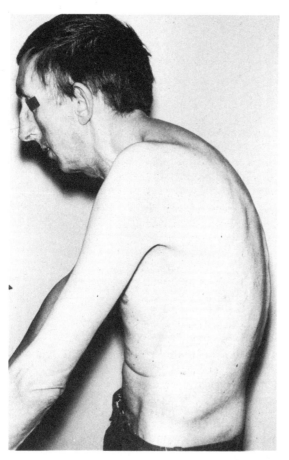

Fig. 7.3. Patient with ankylosing spondylitis showing typical spondylitic posture with loss of the normal spinal curvatures and an exaggerated kyphosis.

be considered. The wrists and shoulders may also be involved but small joints of the hands and feet are only rarely affected in contradistinction to rheumatoid arthritis. Swelling, pain and tenderness over the sternoclavicular, manubriosternal joints and the pubic symphysis are common.

Extra-articular musculoskeletal symptoms also occur. Pain around the heels causing considerable difficulty in walking can be due to either an enthesopathy at the calcaneal insertion of the plantar fascia (*plantar fasciitis*) or the Achilles tendon (*Achilles tendinitis*), or both. It can be a presenting feature. Tenderness over the iliac crests, ischial tuberosities, lower rib margins and greater trochanters can also be found. A *systemic upset* with fever, sweating and weight loss may occur during acute exacerbations of the disease.

Examination

Early in the disease examination of the spine is often unrewarding. Loss of lateral flexion of the lumbar spine is the earliest objective sign of spinal involvement. During phases of sacro-iliitis, tenderness may be elicited by percussing over the sacro-iliac joints. A more sensitive sign is pain resulting from springing the pelvis (*see* Chapter 14). As the spine becomes progressively involved, movements become increasingly restricted. Several methods have been designed to measure spinal restriction. One such is to measure the distance from the floor to the finger tips with the patient attempting to 'touch his toes'. This, like many other methods, is fairly crude and unreliable. A rapid and sensitive test to assess lumbar spine involvement is Schober's test (*see* Chapter 14). In a rigid spine forward flexion is achieved at the hip joint. Measuring chest expansion is one of the more objective signs in the disease. It should be measured at the fourth intercostal space and an average of three readings should be taken.

Examination of peripheral joints may reveal synovitis and/or restriction of movement and careful assessment of all peripheral joints is mandatory, particularly the hips, as early signs of contracture must be treated enthusiastically if permanent deformity is to be avoided. This is particularly true of the juvenile form of the disease (*see* Chapter 12).

◀ Early loss of *lateral* flexion of lumbar spine.

◀ 'Spring' sacro-iliac joints to detect sacro-iliitis.

◀ In rigid spine forward flexion occurs at the *hips*.

Tenderness over the entheses, particularly around the heels, must also be sought.

Complications

Cardiovascular disease
Approximately 4% of patients with ankylosing spondylitis develop lone *aortic incompetence* secondary to non-specific aortitis at the root of the aorta. It usually occurs in patients with longstanding spinal disease. Other cardiac abnormalities such as *conduction defects*, cardiomyopathy and pericarditis have been reported but are rare.

◄ Lone aortic incompetence is due to a non-specific aortitis.

Pulmonary disease
Apical fibrosis and cavitation can complicate ankylosing spondylitis and radiologically mimic pulmonary tuberculosis. The cavities may become secondarily infected with aspergillosis. The cause is unknown. Despite marked limitation of chest expansion, the majority of patients have normal pulmonary function although some demonstrate a mild restrictive ventilatory pattern.

◄ Apical fibrosis and cavitation can mimic TB.

Iritis (uveitis, iridocyclitis)
This is the most common extra-articular manifestation of the disease and affects approximately 20% of patients and often precedes spinal symptoms. It has a temporal association with the peripheral arthritis but not with the spondylitis. The iris and the ciliary body form the anterior part of the uveal tract and inflammation within it is termed *anterior uveitis*, or iridocyclitis or more simply iritis. Enquiries should always be made for symptoms of painful red eyes and photophobia occurring at any time during the course of the disease. Attacks of iritis should be treated vigorously with topical steroids to avoid such complications as synechiae formation (fibrous bands between the iris, the lens and the cornea) which can result in secondary glaucoma and blindness. Intraocular steroid injections are sometimes necessary to settle severe attacks of iritis and expert ophthalmological help should always be sought in monitoring these cases.

◄ Iritis can be a presenting feature — common.

Neurological complications
These are rare. Nerve root irritation (radiculitis) can occur as the nerves run over the inflamed sacro-iliac

joints and give rise to symptoms of classic sciatica. Referred pain from the sacro-iliac joints is more common and has a similar distribution but never extends below the knees. Surprisingly, cases of tetraplegia due to subluxation at the atlanto-axial joint have been reported. Spinal cord damage may also result from traumatic fractures of the rigid spine at any spinal level but the neck is particularly vulnerable and advice about suitable car head restraints and seat-belts should always be given to patients.

Amyloidosis
This is a rare complication of longstanding disease but can lead to renal failure.

Investigations

Laboratory tests
1. The *ESR* is raised during acute phases of the disease as is the plasma viscosity.
2. A *mild leucocytosis* occurs. A normochromic, normocytic anaemia may develop as the disease becomes chronic.
3. Rheumatoid factors are absent from the serum and the *sheep cell agglutination* and *latex tests* are *negative*.
4. *Gammaglobulin levels* may be raised.
5. *HLA* typing shows the presence of B27 in 96% of patients but the test should not be used diagnostically as only a small proportion of B27-positive individuals develop the disease.

◀ HLA typing should be used as a routine diagnostic test.

Radiology
A definite diagnosis of ankylosing spondylitis cannot be made in the absence of radiological signs of bilateral sacro-iliitis. These comprise erosive changes at the joint margins occurring in the lower third of the joints initially, an apparent widening of the 'joint space' is sometimes seen, and juxta-articular sclerosis is seen on both sides of the joint (*Fig.* 7.4). As these changes progress to involve the whole joint, ankylosis occurs and occasionally the original joint line can be seen as a 'ghost' criss-crossed by bony trabeculae. As the disease extends up the spine the characteristic syndesmophyte formation can be seen on lateral and AP

◀ Syndesmophytes are seen earliest at the thoracolumbar junction.

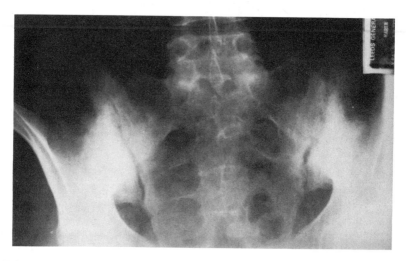

Fig. 7.4. Radiograph showing early changes of sacro-iliitis. Note juxta-articular sclerosis and erosive changes.

lumbar spine films (*see Fig.* 7.2). The posterior facet (apophyseal) joints become sclerotic and eventually ankylosed. Total spine involvement with ankylosis results in the classic appearance of the bamboo spine (*Fig.* 7.5). Radiological evidence of enthesopathy in the form of erosions, sclerosis and soft-tissue calcification should be sought around the ischial tuberosities, greater trochanters, iliac crests, calcanea and patellae. The pubic symphysis can also undergo sclerosis, erosion and ankylosis. Evidence of peripheral joint involvement is usually confined to the hips. The signs are of loss of the radiological joint space, erosions and finally ankylosis in advanced cases.

Treatment and prognosis
As in all chronic rheumatic diseases, once a definite diagnosis has been established the patient should be told and a careful simple explanation of the disease and its implications undertaken.

Physiotherapy
Emphasis in treatment is on *exercise* and the patient should be taught, under the supervision of a

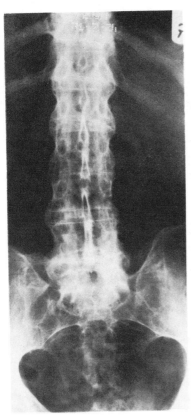

Fig. 7.5. 'Bamboo spine' in longstanding AS. The sacro-iliac joints are ankylosed.

physiotherapist, an exercise programme that should be adhered to daily for the rest of the patient's life. Many physiotherapy departments now undertake regular spondylitic classes during which a group of patients are treated and their progress strictly monitored. This helps maintain patient contact and compliance in the exercise programme. *Hydrotherapy* is a valuable adjunct to dry land exercises and often patients with acute exacerbations respond well to pool therapy.

◀ Regular exercises are the mainstay of treatment programme.

Analgesia

Adequate *analgesia* in the form of anti-inflammatory drugs such as aspirin, naproxen, indomethacin and azapropazone and, if required, phenylbutazone should be given under supervision to allow the patient to exercise through his pain. Inadequacy of anti-inflammatory medication is evidenced by a patient

◀ Use anti-inflammatory drugs to control pain and stiffness to allow patient to exercise.

waking at night with pain or being unable to perform his daily exercises because of pain and stiffness. A nocturnal dose of indomethacin (50 mg) taken with supper is usually adequate in controlling nocturnal pain and early morning stiffness. It may be given in suppository form (100 mg). Oral steroids do not play a part in the anti-inflammatory medication of spondylitics as their response is generally poor and the side-effects far outweigh any clinical benefit.

Radiotherapy

Spinal irradiation, once a popular form of treatment, has now largely been abandoned. Many patients benefited from it but at the cost of an increased malignancy rate, particularly leukaemia, in later life. *Limited radiotherapy* is now reserved for a minority of patients with severe intractable pain unresponsive to standard anti-inflammatory drugs.

◀ Limited radiotherapy is reserved for a few patients with intractable spinal pain.

Surgery

Surgical intervention usually taking the form of hip arthroplasty in those cases with severe hip involvement is often highly successful. Operations to straighten the spinal deformities are fraught with difficulties and can result in irreversible neurological complications and are now rarely performed.

◀ Severe hip involvement may require surgery.

Prognosis

The morbidity of ankylosing spondylitis can be considerable but life expectancy except in severe cases is little changed. The majority of patients are able to maintain a normal life style and, indeed, should be positively encouraged to do so. It is a salutary thought that some people go through life without realizing they have the disease.

Psoriatic arthritis

This is an inflammatory seronegative arthritis affecting some 7% of patients with psoriasis. It can also involve the spine in a way which is indistinguishable from idiopathic ankylosing spondylitis. The sex incidence is determined by the type of psoriatic arthritis. Thus the distal type of arthritis (*see below*) is more common in males whereas females predominate in the other types.

Aetiology

This is unknown. There is strong evidence, however, of a genetic influence in the disease. It is fifty times more common in the families of patients than it is in the normal population. In those patients with concomitant spondylitis and/or sacro-iliitis, there is an increased incidence of tissue type HLA B27 (60–70%).

◄ Genetic influence — 50 times more common in patients' families than in normal population.

Pathology

Psoriatic synovitis can affect any synovial joint and in its early stages is indistinguishable from rheumatoid arthritis. Pannus formation and granulomas, however, are not features but there is usually more fibrosis within the synovium. Ankylosis occurs more frequently in psoriatic arthritis than in rheumatoid disease and a curious periosteal inflammation (periostitis) is common and extends down the shafts of the phalanges causing soft-tissue swelling and tenderness of the digits (sausage-shaped digits, also known as *dactylitis*) (*Fig.* 7.6).

◄ Bony ankylosis and periostitis help distinguish from RA.

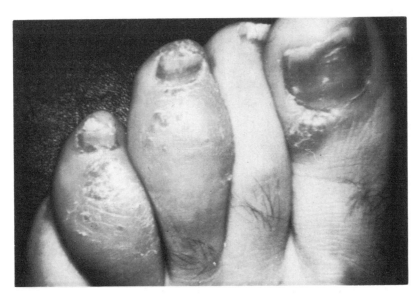

Fig. 7.6. Swollen, tender toes ('dactylitis') in a patient with psoriatic arthritis.

Clinical features

Psoriatic arthritis should always be considered in a patient presenting with any joint pain who has also psoriasis or a family history of psoriasis. The pattern of the arthritis is extremely variable but five subgroups are now recognized:

1. Predominantly distal interphalangeal joint involvement — this is the most common (*Fig. 7.7*).
2. Severe deforming arthritis with occasionally widespread ankylosis — psoriatic arthritis mutilans. This form is rare.
3. A form indistinguishable from rheumatoid arthritis but persistently seronegative for rheumatoid factor and following a more benign course.
4. Oligo- (or mono-) arthritis distributed in an asymmetrical fashion.
5. Spondylitis, associated with any of the above groups or existing alone, may be indistinguishable from idiopathic ankylosing spondylitis. It can, however, be restricted to sacro-iliitis or cervical spondylitis.

Psoriasis usually antedates the onset of the arthritis but occasionally the reverse is true. The skin lesions can be minimal and a search behind the ears, in the scalp, in the umbilicus and natal cleft should

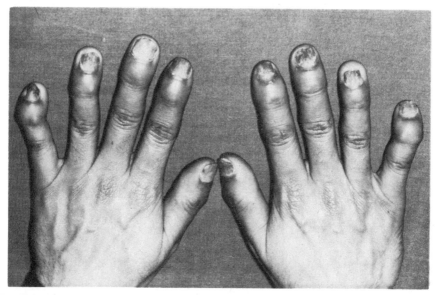

Fig. 7.7. Hands of a patient with typical distal joint with psoriatic arthritis. Note nail dystrophy.

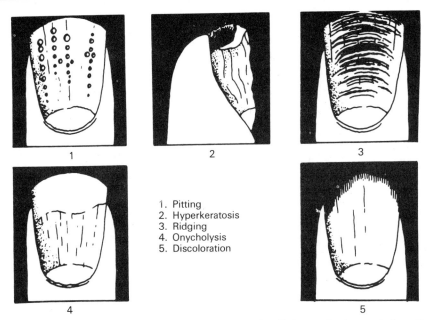

1. Pitting
2. Hyperkeratosis
3. Ridging
4. Onycholysis
5. Discoloration

Fig. 7.8. Drawings illustrating the various forms of nail dystrophy in psoriatic arthritis (*from* Wright, V. (1979) *Scand. J. Rheumatol.* Suppl. 32).

be made as well as in the more usual places such as at the elbows, knees and on the trunk. The nail dystrophy of psoriasis (*see Fig.* 7.7) consisting of pitting, ridging, hyperkeratosis and onycholysis (separation of the nail from the nail bed) (*Fig.* 7.8) has a much closer relationship to the arthritis than do the skin lesions and, indeed, may be the only manifestation of the disease. A curious phenomenon seen in some patients is the juxtaposition of psoriatic nail(s) and an arthritic distal interphalangeal joint(s). The reasons for this 'geographical' association are obscure. The mutilating form of the arthritis is usually associated with extensive skin psoriasis but in the other types the severity of the psoriasis has no relationship to the severity of the arthritis. The arthritis can present chiefly as a monoarthritis, usually of the knees but other large joints may be affected initially. A more comon mode of presentation is insidiously with involvement of the small joints of the hands and feet often in an asymmetrical fashion and associated with early morning exacerbations as in rheumatoid arthritis.

Enquiry about back pain, with a typical spondylitic early morning stiffness, should always be made and appropriate radiographs (AP pelvis and cervical

◀ Nail dystrophy closely associated with arthritis.

◀ A history of back pain (due to spondylitis) should always be sought.

spine) taken, otherwise psoriatic spondylitis will be missed and the patient run the risk of permanent spinal deformities which otherwise might have been avoided.

Differential diagnosis

Not all patients with psoriasis and an arthritis have psoriatic arthritis. Psoriasis and rheumatoid arthritis are both common conditions and occasionally will coexist. Tests for rheumatoid factor will resolve the issue if they are positive, as will the presence of rheumatoid nodules. The few patients with persistently seronegative rheumatoid disease (probably less than 5%) will, however, continue to cause confusion. Radiological examination may or may not be helpful in these cases (*see below*). If sacro-iliitis is also present then the diagnosis is much more likely to be psoriatic arthritis as sacro-iliac joint involvement in rheumatoid disease is rare. *Gout* may also cause diagnostic confusion being a seronegative asymmetrical arthritis but crystal analysis of the synovial fluid, if available, will show typical negatively birefringent needle-like crystals of sodium urate (*see* Chapter 8). Serum uric acid levels are an unreliable diagnostic discriminator as they can be elevated in psoriasis and may be normal in acute gout.

◀ RA and psoriasis may coexist and give rise to diagnostic confusion.

◀ Rheumatoid nodules are not a feature of psoriatic arthritis.

◀ Pelvic radiographs may reveal sacro-iliitis.

Extra-articular features

Extra-articular features are rare in psoriatic arthritis but conjunctivitis, iritis and even keratoconjunctivitis sicca do occur. Other features such as spondylitic aortic valve disease and amyloid deposition have been described.

◀ Extra-articular features as for AS — but rarer.

Investigations

Laboratory tests

1. The ESR and plasma viscosity are elevated in acute attacks but may also be elevated during severe exacerbation of the skin lesions.
2. A mild neutrophilia is not uncommon.
3. A rise in gammaglobulins (particularly IgA) is often seen.

4. Tests for rheumatoid factor are negative.
5. A mild normochromic, normocytic anaemia is seen in chronic disease.
6. Synovial fluid analysis shows an inflammatory fluid with a high cell count (mainly neutrophils) and complement levels in the fluid are usually normal — unlike rheumatoid arthritis when synovial fluid complement levels are depressed.

Radiology
No one radiological feature is specific to psoriatic arthritis and it can mimic rheumatoid disease or gout, but typical lesions and the distribution of the arthritis can provide important diagnostic clues. There is emphasis on asymmetrical erosive changes in the distal interphalangeal joints and a relative sparing of the metacarpophalangeal joints. Subperiosteal new bone formation in the phalanges reflects the periostitis and erosions well away from the joint margins are sometimes observed. Periarticular bone destruction sometimes leading to complete dissolution of bone, particularly in the distal phalanges, is a significant feature of psoriatic arthritis. A characteristic whittling of the distal bone ends of the phalanges with associated cupping of the proximal ends leads to a *'pencil-in-cup'* appearance (*Fig. 7.9*). Joint ankylosis is also more common than in rheumatoid arthritis and changes of ankylosing spondylitis may be seen in the spine.

◀ Asymmetrical erosive changes seen radiographically

◀ Peripheral joint ankylosis.
◀ Changes of ankylosing spondylitis may be seen in the spine.

Treatment and prognosis
Fortunately, most patients respond to standard non-steroidal anti-inflammatory medications such as aspirin, indomethacin, naproxen or azapropazone and their arthritis remains mild. In those patients with more aggressive arthritis other agents such as gold (administered in the same way as in rheumatoid disease) and immunosuppressive agents, e.g. methotrexate and azathioprine, may have to be resorted to. Unfortunately the response to all these agents is unpredictable and inconsistent. Penicillamine does not work. Occasionally corticosteroids may be required to control symptoms. *Joint aspiration* and intra-articular corticosteroids can often prove beneficial and allow physiotherapists to mobilize an otherwise compromised joint.

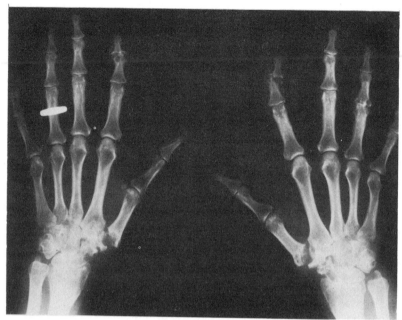

Fig. 7.9. Radiograph of hands of patient with psoriatic arthritis. Note erosive changes in DIP joints and 'whittling' of middle phalanx of the right index finger. Both carpi are involved but there is sparing of the MCP joints.

Physiotherapy is again a vital part of any treatment regime for psoriatic arthritis, particularly in those patients with associated spondylitis. Unfortunately very little can be done to arrest the course of psoriatic arthritis mutilans; however, it is amazing how much useful function can be preserved in severely deformed hands.

Reiter's disease

This is a symptom triad often referred to as Reiter's syndrome comprising:
1. A seronegative arthritis affecting the lower limbs predominantly
2. Conjunctivitis
3. Non-specific urethritis

The first description of the disease dates from the 16th century but the eponymous title, Reiter's disease, was earned by Hans Reiter in 1916 for his report of a patient who developed conjunctivitis, arthritis and a urethral discharge following an attack of dysentery. Since then two forms of the disease have been recognized, namely *genital* (or venereal) usually following promiscuous sexual exposure, and *intestinal*, usually following an attack of bacillary (shigella) dysentery.

The overall incidence of the disease is unknown, but the dysenteric form is more common in Scandinavian countries whilst the venereal form is more common in this country. One of the major problems in assessing prevalence is the lack of uniformity of diagnostic criteria for the disease. Many authorities now accept the diagnosis of Reiter's disease without the full triad of symptoms and the presence of an acute arthritis and non-specific urethritis is generally accepted as being sufficient for the diagnosis in the correct clinical setting. Conjunctivitis is the most variable and transitory of the triad and is often missed by both patient and physician. Objective evidence of a non-specific urethritis is also notoriously difficult to obtain. Symptoms may be minimized and go unnoticed and usually amount to no more than transient dysuria and a slight penile discharge. It is thought that about 2% of patients with non-specific non-gonococcal urethritis attending clinics for sexually acquired disease in the UK develop Reiter's disease.

The disease is much more common in young males than females (sex ratio 20 : 1) but this may in part be due to difficulty in making a diagnosis of urethritis in the female as it is more often symptomless. A transient seronegative oligoarthritis in a young male should always arouse a suspicion of Reiter's disease and prompt enquiry about change in bowel habit or symptoms of urethritis.

◀ Two forms of disease, venereal (genital) and dysenteric (intestinal).

◀ 2% of patients with non-specific urethritis develop Reiter's disease.

Aetiology
It is likely that Reiter's disease is a generalized reaction to an infection, either urogenital or intestinal. In this respect the arthritis can be regarded as a *reactive arthritis* (*see below*).

The dysenteric form follows infection by *Shigella flexneri*, *Shigella dysenteriae* and sometimes salmonellae. *Yersinia enterocolitica* has also been implicated, especially in Scandinavia. The syndrome not uncommonly follows non-specific diarrhoea when no infective organism can be isolated.

The causative organism(s) in the genital type is as yet unidentified but *Chlamydia trachomatis* seems a likely candidate. It is found in up to 50% of patients with non-specific urethritis and rising antibody titres to the organism are found in patients with Reiter's disease but not in those with non-specific urethritis alone.

Why some patients exposed to these infections should develop Reiter's disease and others do not is almost certainly genetically determined. It has been shown that between 63% and 90% of patients with Reiter's disease carry the tissue antigen B27 in contrast to 9% with uncomplicated non-specific urethritis and 6% of controls. In addition to this a family study conducted in this country showed an increased prevalence of sacro-iliitis, spondylitis and psoriasis in the relatives of patients with Reiter's disease. This latter finding has helped place Reiter's disease firmly in the spondarthritic group.

◀ 60–90% of patients carry HLA B27.

◀ Increased prevalence of psoriasis and spondylitis in relatives of patients with Reiter's disease.

Clinical manifestations

The classic presentation of Reiter's disease is of a young man with an acute oligoarthritis usually of the knee, conjunctivitis and non-specific urethritis occurring some 1–4 weeks after sexual exposure (usually, although not necessarily, promiscuous) or an attack of dysentery.

The arthritis

The most commonly affected joint is the knee. The arthritis is usually self-limiting and often transitory lasting no more than 2 or 3 days. It can, however, be acute causing tense effusions and even knee joint rupture. Asymmetrical oligo- or even polyarthritis can occur and develop into a chronic relapsing, destructive arthropathy particularly of the knees and forefeet. It may eventually be indistinguishable from psoriatic arthritis. Further attacks of arthritis are not necessarily associated with further episodes of urethritis. Spinal involvement occurs in about 20% of cases, the majority of which will be B27 positive. Sacro-iliitis is the most comon manifestation and can be unilateral. Spondylitis also occurs but it is usually confined to the lumbar region and rarely extends to produce a bamboo spine. Enthesopathies, identical to those seen in ankylosing spondylitis, are not uncommon, the site of predilection being the heels.

◀ Knee is most commonly involved joint.

◀ Spinal involvement in 20% of cases — majority B27 positive.

Periostitis as in psoriatic arthritis affects the shafts of the phalanges and leads to typical tender sausage-shaped digits.

Ocular lesions

The conjunctivitis is often mild and may go unnoticed. It is sometimes associated with a sterile discharge which usually settles after 1–4 weeks. Occasionally corneal ulceration, keratitis and episcleritis may supervene. Uveitis also occurs in the acute stages of the disease and is much more common in patients with relapsing arthritis, affecting approximately 30%. This figure approaches 50% in those patients with sacro-iliitis. Intraocular haemorrhages and retrobulbar neuritis have been reported but are very rare.

Urethritis

Symptoms may be minimal. Mild dysuria with/or without a clear discharge is often ignored or forgotten by the patient and careful history taking is essential if this vital clue is not to be missed. In a few cases the discharge is more florid and acute haemorrhagic cystitis does occur. Objective evidence of urethritis should always be sought. The time-honoured 'two-glass test' is still a useful bedside technique. The patient is asked to void the initial portion of an early morning urine stream into one glass and then the remainder of the stream into another glass. If urethritis is present, and sufficiently severe, the initial urine will contain pus cells, red cells and filaments which will be absent or less concentrated in the second specimen. A more reliable method is to take a deep urethral swab prior to micturition and to examine a smear microscopically for pus cells and culture it for infection (particularly to rule out a concomitant gonococcal infection).

Mucocutaneous lesions

These are not necessary for the diagnosis but can often be important contributory factors. The most characteristic of these lesions is *keratodermia blenorrhagica*. This occurs usually on the soles (*Fig.* 7.10) but can be seen on the palms and in a few cases spreads to involve the trunk and scalp but rarely the face. The initial lesion is a brown macule which progresses to form a sterile pustule and becomes scaly. The lesions are indistinguishable from pustu-

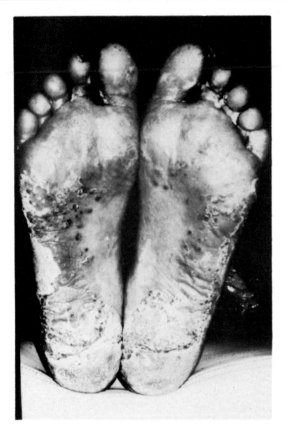

Fig. 7.10. Keratodermia blenorrhagica on the soles of a patient with Reiter's disease.

lar psoriasis both clinically and histologically. Nail changes sometimes occur in relationship to keratodermia and these, too, are indistinguishable from the nail dystrophy seen in psoriasis. Nail shedding is not uncommon.

Shallow coalescing ulcers with a serpiginous border may affect the glans penis. They are usually painless and are called *circinate balanitis*. Similar lesions may also affect the buccal mucosa. A pharyngitis also occurs. The mucocutaneous lesions tend to be associated with more aggressive arthritis.

◀ Circinate balanitis occurs on the glans penis.

Other clinical manifestations
Systemic upset with fever, malaise and weight loss often occurs. Rarer complications are pericarditis, myocarditis, aortitis indistinguishable from that seen in ankylosing spondylitis, and cardiac conduction

◀ There may be systemic upset.

defects. Pleurisy also occurs and amyloidosis has been reported. A variety of neurological symptoms, including meningoencephalitis and transient hemiplegia, occur in 1% of patients.

Investigations
1. ESR and plasma viscosity are elevated during active phases of the disease and can reach very high sustained values.
2. Polymorpholeucocytosis can be marked.
3. Patients with chronic relapsing disease develop a normochromic, normocytic anaemia.
4. Hypergammaglobulinaemia is often detected.
5. Rheumatoid factors are absent from the serum.
6. Synovial fluid analysis reveals an acute inflammatory, sterile fluid with a high cell content (mainly neutrophils) and low viscosity.

Radiology
In the majority of self-limiting cases, radiological changes are confined to soft-tissue swelling around affected joints. The radiological changes seen in chronic arthritis are similar to those of psoriatic arthritis with cartilage loss and erosions. Spinal changes mimic those of ankylosing spondylitis but the sacro-iliitis is not uncommonly unilateral and syndesmophyte formation is not as marked and also tends to be asymmetrical as in psoriatic spondylitis. The bamboo spine is a rare finding in Reiter's disease. Calcaneal spurs occurring as a result of an enthesopathy of the plantar fascia are seen as a fluffy spike of calcification in the plantar fascia just anterior to the antero-inferior border of the calcaneum.

◄ Peripheral joint changes may be similar to those of psoriatic arthritis.

◄ 'Fluffy' calcaneal spurs common.

Treatment
In most cases, the arthritis is self-limiting, and treatment is in the main, purely symptomatic.

Analgesia
Non-steroidal anti-inflammatory drugs are used in the same way as for any other arthritis. Indocid, if it can be tolerated, is the drug of choice, although aspirin, naproxen and azapropazone may be equally effective in some patients. Local joint aspiration and injection with corticosteroids can prove invaluable in the more severe cases.

Physiotherapy
Physiotherapy aimed at maintaining muscle function is important, particularly when the knee joint is involved as quadriceps wasting can occur with surprising rapidity. Spinal exercises are vital for those patients with spondylitis. Plantar fasciitis can be particularly troublesome in this condition. Local steroid injections may be tried in conjunction with shock-absorbing heel pads, and a course of ultrasound. If this proves unsuccessful and the condition becomes chronic, local irradiation to the painful area is often helpful.

Treatment of urethritis and conjunctivitis
The urethritis always responds to either erythromycin or tetracycline, although neither of these antibiotics influences the musculoskeletal symptoms of the disease, even when the urethritis is cured. Iritis is treated with topical steroids but the sterile conjunctivitis rarely requires treatment but, if severe, steroid drops should be used.

◄ Antibiotic treatment of the urethritis does not influence the arthritis.

Immunosuppression
In patients with chronic relapsing arthritis associated with keratodermia blenorrhagica, methotrexate is sometimes of value in controlling both the skin lesions and the arthritis but success is, unfortunately, unpredictable. Intramuscular adrenocorticotrophic hormone can be used in difficult cases but again response is variable as it is to oral corticosteroids.

Enteropathic arthritis
This group of arthritides is characterized by an association either with bowel disease, inflammatory or infective, or with intestinal bypass operations performed for obesity. The chief members of this group are the arthritis associated with *ulcerative colitis* and *Crohn's disease*, in both of which an increased frequency of ankylosing spondylitis is also seen.

Enteritis caused by salmonella, *Yersinia enterocolitica* and possibly other gut infections can also trigger an arthritis in susceptible individuals. This has often been regarded as a 'reactive arthritis' in much the same way as rheumatic fever or postviral arthritis. However, many authorities now believe that arthritis associated with gut infection is a variant of Reiter's disease.

Another much rarer member of this group is *Whipple's disease* (intestinal lipodystrophy) which can also be complicated by a peripheral arthritis and is described briefly below.

Aetiology

This is unknown. One attractive theory is that antigens contained within the bowel lumen escape across the bowel mucosa, which may be damaged in some way, and enter the circulation to form antigen–antibody complexes which can enter the joints and stimulate a synovitis. There is evidence in ulcerative colitis that bacterial antigens normally confined to the lumen do cross into the circulation, but as yet no complexes containing such antigens have been found within the joints of patients with colitic arthritis. In patients with morbid obesity who undergo intestinal bypass operations to decrease food absorption, a peripheral arthritis can develop which is abolished when the normal bowel anatomy is restored. Similarly in ulcerative colitis the arthropathy can be abolished by resection of the diseased segment of bowel. Both these facts suggest that absorption of bowel antigens into the circulation is important in stimulating arthritis and also in its chronicity.

◄ Restoration of bowel anatomy in 'bypass' arthritis is curative.

Individuals possessing B27 are more prone to developing reactive arthritis after enteritis but there is no relationship between the possession of B27 and the peripheral arthritis of ulcerative colitis and Crohn's disease. However, in patients with these conditions who develop ankylosing spondylitis there is an increased frequency of HLA B27 although it is not as high as it is in idiopathic spondylitis. In addition to this there is an increased prevalence of ulcerative colitis in those families of patients with ankylosing spondylitis.

◄ Patients possessing HLA B27 are more prone to enteropathic arthritis.

Arthritis associated with ulcerative colitis

Arthritis can occur in association with ulcerative colitis at any stage of the disease but it is more common in the first 5 years and can antedate the onset of bowel symptoms although it is usually seen during acute exacerbations of the colitis. It affects approximately 10% of patients and the sex ratio is equal. The most common presentation is as a

◄ Arthritis may antedate colitis.

monoarthritis usually of the knee but a polyarthritis involving knees, elbows, shoulders and small joints of the hands and feet, in an asymmetrical fashion, does occur. When the colitis settles, the arthritis always goes into remission and settles without any sequelae. Patients with more extensive gut involvement are more likely to develop the arthritis. Occasionally the arthritis can be so severe as to warrant removal of the diseased bowel which always results in abolition of the arthritis.

◀ When colitis settles arthritis remits.

Ankylosing spondylitis occurs in approximately 6% of patients and is not related to colitic activity and is not influenced by resection of the diseased bowel. Clinically it resembles idiopathic ankylosing spondylitis. Interestingly 14% of patients with ulcerative colitis have asymptomatic sacro-iliitis without spondylitis.

◀ Ankylosing spondylitis occurs in 6% of patients — sacro-iliitis in 14%.

Erythema nodosum occurring during acute attacks of ulcerative colitis is sometimes also associated with the arthritis. *Clubbing* is well recognized and a periosteal reaction, not unlike that seen in hypertrophic pulmonary osteoarthropathy (*see* Chapter 11), giving rise to subperiosteal new bone formation and tenderness around the ankles and wrists, has been described. *Uveitis* also occurs.

Investigations

Laboratory tests
There are no diagnostic laboratory tests. The ESR and plasma viscosity are elevated and tests for rheumatoid factor are negative. Synovial fluid analysis and synovial histology show the changes of acute inflammation and are also non-specific.

Radiology
This is also unhelpful diagnostically except in patients with associated ankylosing spondylitis and sacro-iliitis. The sacro-iliac joint changes can often be detected on the barium studies used to investigate the bowel disease. The radiological changes are identical to those seen in idiopathic ankylosing spondylitis.

Treatment
In the majority of cases the peripheral arthritis is short-lived but can be extremely painful. *Non-steroidal anti-inflammatory drugs* are exhibited in the usual way provided they can be tolerated. There

is no evidence that they have any adverse effect on the colitis. The most effective way of treating the arthritis long term is to bring the bowel disease under control. Occasionally this necessitates the use of *corticosteroids*, either topically as enemas or systemically. Sulphasalazine is used for more long-term control. Local joint aspiration and injection of corticosteroids are also very effective. Physiotherapy is important to maintain muscle power and prevent contractures.

◄ Definitive treatment of the arthritis (but not spondylitis) is to control the colitis.

Arthritis associated with Crohn's disease (regional enteritis)
This is for the most part identical to the arthritis seen in patients with ulcerative colitis and can also be associated with asymptomatic sacro-iliitis and ankylosing spondylitis. However, the following important differences should be noted:
1. The arthritis is not influenced by reaction of the diseased segment of bowel. This is probably because Crohn's disease can affect many different parts of the bowel at the same time.
2. The arthritis shows a weaker association with exacerbations of the bowel disease than does ulcerative colitic arthropathy.
3. Synovial histology may reveal granulomatous lesions similar to those found in the gut.
   Treatment is as for ulcerative colitic arthropathy.

Whipple's disease (intestinal lipodystrophy)
This is a rare condition chiefly affecting males. It results from infection of the small bowel and leads to *malabsorption* and profound weight loss. Other features are *lymphadenopathy* and a migratory *polyarthritis* which is often a presenting feature and is seen in up to 60% of patients. *Sacro-iliitis* has been described in association with Whipple's disease and even ankylosing spondylitis has been reported. Hence the tentative inclusion of this disease in the seronegative spondarthritides. Diagnosis depends on the identification of periodic-acid-Schiff (PAS) positive material (probably bacterial in origin) in the macrophages of the small intestinal mucosa obtained by jejunal biopsy. Similar PAS-positive material has been identified in the synovial macrophages of the affected joints.

Both the arthritis and the malabsorption respond to treatment with antibiotics, the most usual one being tetracycline although lincomycin is also used. The response is usually good but a few patients show a late relapse. Left untreated the disease is fatal.

Enteric arthropathy

This group of arthropathies has already been alluded to in the introductory section. The most common organisms involved are *salmonella, shigella* (also responsible for Reiter's disease) and *yersinia*. It has also been reported in antibiotic-induced *pseudomembranous colitis* and non-specific diarrhoea.

The arthritis is usually an acute *mono-* or *oligoarthritis* affecting large peripheral joints especially the *knee*. It appears about 4 weeks after the onset of the enteric infection and in the majority of cases settles within a month, though it can persist for as long as a year or more. Many authorities believe this form of arthritis to be a 'forme fruste' of Reiter's disease without the urethritis and conjunctivitis.

Treatment is purely symptomatic with anti-inflammatory drugs. Antibiotic treatment is usually not necessary for the enteritis, though occasionally frank *infective arthritis* can occur with *salmonella* infections. These organisms can also be responsible for osteomyelitis and both these clinical situations demand the use of high-dose systemic antibiotics for successful outcome.

◀ Salmonella enteritis may cause a frank infective arthritis.

Behçet's syndrome

The inclusion of Behçet's syndrome in the seronegative spondarthritis group is still speculative and its aetiology is unknown. It is a symptom complex comprising *arthritis, iritis* and *recurrent oral* and *genital ulceration*. The most constant feature is aphthous-type oral ulceration. Other features are:

◀ Behçet's syndrome:
● arthritis
● iritis (uveitis)
● orogenital ulceration

1. Peripheral synovitis which is asymmetrical and seronegative (60% of cases)
2. Vasculitis (including erythema nodosum) and thrombophlebitis
3. Septic skin lesions occurring on the arms, legs and chest (30% of cases)
4. Meningitis and meningo-encephalitis (rare)
5. Sacro-iliitis and ankylosing spondylitis (rare), probably B27 associated

6. Pericarditis (rare)

It is more common in countries bordering on the eastern Mediterranean and also in Japan. The original cases in Turkey were described by Behçet and it still remains a common disease in that country. Males are affected more frequently than females. The disease follows a course of relapses and remissions. The oral and genital ulceration can be extremely painful. Oral ulcers have many features of simple aphthous ulceration but they tend to be more marked and extend down into the pharynx causing severe dysphagia. They usually heal within 2–3 weeks, sometimes with scarring. Asymptomatic vaginal ulcers are not uncommon and are discovered on routine speculum examination. Sometimes they are associated with a discharge and when the ulceration occurs on the vulva this can lead to severe dyspareunia. In the male, the ulcers tend to be restricted to the scrotum and shaft of the penis. The arthritis is mild and self-limiting and usually affects the knees and ankles. A recurrent *uveitis* can be very severe and result in blindness if it affects the posterior uveal tract and extends into the retina and vitreous. Uveitis of the anterior uveal tract can result in synechiae and hypopyon — pus in the anterior chamber. Uveitis is often bilateral but only rarely is it an initial manifestation of the disease and occurs in some 60% of cases.

◀ Recurrent uveitis can lead to blindness.

Treatment

Treatment of the oral/genital ulcers is purely symptomatic. Local anaesthetic creams are used and corticosteroid pellets applied directly to the oral ulcers can be very effective. Systemic steroids are of limited value and their long-term use is not justified. Immunosuppressive agents such as methotrexate and azathioprine are also disappointing in their effect though some patients with particularly active and frequently recurrent disease do gain benefit. Chlorambucil has been claimed to be of benefit for those patients with sight-threatening uveitis. Fortunately topical and intra-ocular steroids control most patients during acute attacks of uveitis.

The arthritis tends to be the least troublesome of the complications. It is self-limiting and responds well to non-steroidal anti-inflammatory drugs and/or intra-articular steroids.

Further Reading

Moll J. M. H. (ed.) (1980) *Ankylosing Spondylitis.*
Edinburgh, Churchill Livingstone.
Wright V. and Moll J. M. H. (ed.) (1976) *Sero-negative
Polyarthritis.* Amsterdam, North-Holland.

Crystal-induced arthritis   **8**

A variety of crystals are found in synovial fluid but not all result in an acute arthritis. Two types of crystal which are known to be directly implicated in acute arthritis and joint destruction are *sodium urate* and *calcium pyrophosphate dihydrate* (CPPD) occurring in *gout* and *pseudogout* (pyrophosphate arthropathy) respectively, and it is these two forms of arthritis that concern us in this chapter.

Identification of crystals in synovial fluid
Routine microscopy of synovial fluid in gout and pseudogout will often reveal crystals though their characterization on purely morphological grounds can be extremely difficult. As a general rule the crystals of sodium urate are long, thin and needle-like whilst those of CPPD tend to be shorter and fatter. In order for a more positive identification to be made, the fluid should be viewed under polarized light on a *polarizing light microscope*. Such a microscope has two polarizing filters — one below (*the polarizer*) and one above (*the analyser*) — with a rotating stage, and orientated in such a way that their planes of polarization are at right-angles, i.e. *crossed polars*. Because the planes of polarization are at right-angles no light will reach the eye-piece unless an object capable of altering the plane of polarization of the light is placed on the stage. Sodium urate and CPPD are both crystals which have this optical property. They are *birefringent*. When viewed under a polarizing microscope such crystals will appear bright at certain positions as their long axis is rotated through 360° and conversely there will be certain positions when no light will be transmitted. The angle between the long axis of the

crystal and the plane of polarization at which extinction of light occurs is known as the *angle of extinction* of the crystal. In the case of urate this occurs when a crystal is parallel to the plane of polarization of either the polarizer or the analyser. This is known as *negative birefringence* — thus sodium urate crystals are *negatively birefringent*. In the case of CPPD crystals the angle of extinction is oblique to the plane of polarized light. This is known as *positive birefringence* — thus CPPD crystals are *positively birefringent* (though only weakly so). The optical properties of these two crystals are thus vital for accurate identification and an important aid to the diagnosis of gout and pseudogout.

◀ Sodium urate crystals are negatively birefringent, calcium pyrophosphate crystals positively birefringent.

Gout

This is a systemic disease resulting from the precipitation of crystals of sodium urate from the body fluids into many soft tissues, including synovial membranes where they induce an intense and often destructive arthritis — *gouty arthritis*.

Aetiology

Sodium urate is a salt of uric acid. Uric acid is the final breakdown product of *purine* metabolism in man. Purine bases (*adenine, guanine*) are essential for energy transfer reactions and in the synthesis of nucleic acids in all cells. The synthetic and degradation pathways of purine metabolism are shown in *Fig.* 8.1 in a simplified form. Man has no means of further metabolizing uric acid as he lacks the enzyme uricase which is possessed by most other mammalian species. He is dependent for its elimination on *renal excretion* and to a lesser extent on its *bacterial degradation* in the gut (*uricolysis*). Both these methods are relatively inefficient. In the kidney uric acid passes freely into the glomerular filtrate and is then completely resorbed in the proximal tubule only to be actively secreted by the distal tubule and voided in the urine (*Fig.* 8.2). The fact that normal serum levels of uric acid (defined as up to 0·42 mmol/l for males and 0·36 mmol/l for females) are very close to its serum solubility product also helps to explain why man is susceptible to gout.

◀ Man lacks the enzyme uricase and depends on renal excretion and urico-lysis in the gut for the elimination of uric acid.

Sex, age and *genetic* constitution are also important factors in determining the concentration of uric

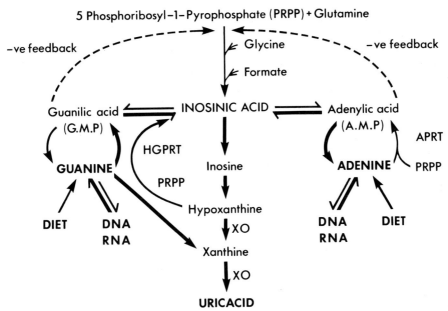

Fig. 8.1. Simplified synthetic and degradation pathways of purine metabolism. HGPRT = hypoxanthine guanine phosphoribosyl transferase; APRT = adenine phosphoribosyl transferase; XO = xanthine oxydase.

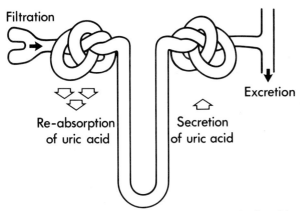

Fig. 8.2. Diagram showing renal handling of uric acid.

acid in the blood. As has already been indicated, the mean level of uric acid is higher in males than it is in females. However, when one studies postmenopausal females the difference becomes less pronounced and female levels approach those of the male. The concentration of uric acid also increases with age, strikingly so until the third decade in men

◀ Concentration of uric acid increases with age.

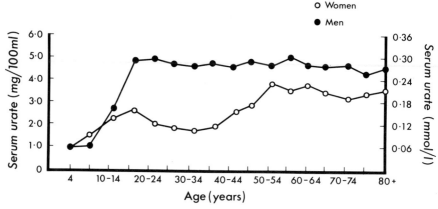

Fig. 8.3. Graph illustrating the effects of sex and age on mean serum urate concentration.

and then stabilizing until the seventh decade when it begins a slower rise (*Fig.* 8.3).

Hyperuricaemia
A rise in the serum uric acid (hyperuricaemia) is a characteristic finding in gout though not all people with hyperuricaemia develop gout. Two basic defects can cause hyperuricaemia, one is *over-production* and the other is *underexcretion of uric acid.* When the cause of this overproduction or under-excretion is known it is called *secondary hyper-uricaemia* (leading to *secondary gout*) but when it is not the condition is known as *essential hyperuricaemia* (leading to *primary gout*). In essential hyper-uricaemia primary overproduction of uric acid can be identified by measuring the uric acid excretion in a 24-hour urine sample in a patient on a purine-free diet, 600 mg (3·6 mmol)/24 h being the upper limit of normal. A simpler method is to measure the urinary uric acid/creatinine ratio after an overnight fast (upper limit of normal 0·54 in adults). Further, in some patients both overproduction and under-excretion are present and identification of these patients is more difficult. In the majority of patients with essential hyperuricaemia underexcretion is thought to be the major factor but as yet undisco-vered enzyme defects, leading to overproduction of uric acid, cannot be ruled out.

◀ Hyperuricaemia does not necessarily lead to gout.

Secondary hyperuricaemia
Secondary hyperuricaemia can be precipitated by any condition resulting either in the *overproduction*

Table 8.1.   Causes of secondary hyperuricaemia

Overproduction of uric acid
1. Increased cell turnover
      Lymphoproliferative disorders, Hodgkin's and other
         lymphomas
      Myeloproliferative disorders, Leukaemia, poly-
         cythaemia rubra vera, myeloma
      Carcinomatosis
      Haemolytic anaemia
      Secondary polycythaemia
      Severe psoriasis
2. Increased dietery intake of purines, e.g. sweetmeats,
      offal
3. Enzyme defects in purine biosynthesis and
      degradation,
      Lesch-Nyhan syndrome (HGPRT deficiency)
      PRPP synthetase overactivity

Decreased renal excretion
1. Renal failure from whatever cause
2. Poisoning/inhibition of renal tubular excretion pathway
      a. Drugs, e.g. *thiazide diuretics*, low-dose salicylates
      b. Lead (saturnine gout)
      c. Acidaemia, e.g. diabetic, ketoacidosis, starvation,
         excessive alcohol, Von Gierke's disease

of *uric acid* or in its *underexcretion* (*Table* 8.1).
Overproduction is seen in conditions causing an
increased nucleic acid degradation often arising from
an increased cell turnover, e.g. *myeloproliferative
disorders*. Underexcretion is common in patients
with renal disease but the most common cause of
secondary hyperuricaemia in this country is the
consumption of *thiazide diuretics*. These drugs
poison the active secretion of uric acid into the renal
tubule. Other drugs, particularly low-dose *salicylates*, have a similar effect. *Alcohol*, by producing a
ketoacidosis, will inhibit tubular secretion and cause
hyperuricaemia. Diabetic ketoacidosis and acidosis
occurring during starvation (especially 'crash' diets)
have the same effect.

◄ The most common
cause of secondary hyper-
uricaemia is thiazide
diuretics.

◄ 'Crash' diets may in-
duce hyperuricaemia.

Enzyme defects. Several of these have now been
identified, all of which can result in hyperuricaemia.
Deficiency of the purine salvage enzyme hypoxanthine guanine phosphoribosyl transferase
(HGPRT) (*see Fig.* 8.1) is a rare X-linked inborn
error of metabolism and results in the *Lesch–Nyhan
syndrome*. This normally manifests itself in child-

hood. Patients develop severe tophaceous gout (*see below*), choreoathetosis and mental deficiency and exhibit a bizarre compulsion to mutilate themselves. Very few survive into adulthood.

Phosphoribosylpyrophosphate synthetase is a key enzyme in the production and regulation of nucleotides. A rare x-linked disorder resulting in its overactivity causes overproduction of purines and uric acid which can result in gout.

In some families with gout there is increased synthesis of *ribose-5-phosphate*, one of the substrates for purine biosynthesis. This leads to excessive amounts of phosphoribosylpyrophosphate and increased purine and uric acid production and hence gout. No specific enzyme defect has yet been discovered in this abnormality.

Patients with *Von Gierke's disease* (glycogen storage disease type 1 — glucose-6-phosphatase deficiency) develop hyperuricaemia and gout provided they survive long enough. These patients suffer a lactic acidosis and ketosis secondary to their impaired carbohydrate metabolism and uric acid excretion is therefore impaired.

Mechanisms involved in acute gouty arthritis

The primary event in an attack of gout is the deposition of monosodium urate crystals in the synovium and synovial fluid. Why sodium urate should precipitate in certain joints and tissues is not entirely understood. One particular anomaly is that in many patients the serum uric acid is normal during an acute attack but concentrations during symptom-free intervals can be very high.

◄ The serum urate concentration may be normal in an acute attack of gout.

The most commonly affected joint is the first metatarsophalangeal joint but any joint, including (rarely) the synovial joints of the spine, can be affected. *Trauma*, changes in *pH* of the joint micro-environment and *temperature* changes have all been implicated as causative factors.

◄ Any joint may be affected by gout, but it is most common in the first metatarsophalangeal joint.

Once sodium urate has been precipitated, the crystals induce an intense inflammatory response in the synovial membrane. Polymorphonuclear leucocytes are then attracted to the inflammatory area by chemotaxis and phagocytose the crystals. In so doing lysosomal membranes within the leucocytes rupture and proteolytic enzymes contained in them are released into the synovial fluid. This increases the inflammatory response and results, after repeated attacks, in cartilage destruction and bony damage (*Fig.* 8.4).

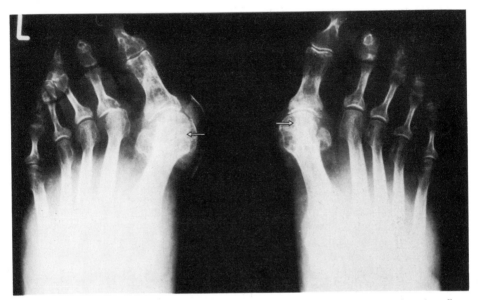

Fig. 8.4. Radiograph of feet showing destructive changes of gout in the first metatarsophalangeal joints and lucent areas in the head of the metatarsals due to tophaceous deposits (arrowed).

Prevalence

Approximately 0·03% of the European population will suffer an attack of gout. A much higher prevalence is found in those ethnic groups who have a high incidence of hyperuricaemia. Such groups are the Maoris of New Zealand and other Polynesian races. Males above the age of 40 are the most commonly affected and it is extremely rare for a premenopausal female to suffer from primary gout. If such a patient presents then one should always suspect one of the causes of secondary gout listed in *Table* 8.1.

◀ Gout in a pre-menopausal female is very rare.

Dietary factors

Dietary factors rarely cause gout, contrary to popular belief. However, a high alcohol intake by inducing a lactic acidosis and urate retention by the kidney will precipitate gouty attacks in predisposed individuals. Occasionally the consumption of a diet with a high purine content (e.g. sweetbreads and offal) will have the same result. It has been suggested that the increased prevalence of gout in some areas is due to the higher lead content in the environment, especially drinking water. Lead poisons the renal excretion of urate and the gout that results is known as *saturnine gout*.

Genetic factors

A family history of gout is not uncommon but estimates of the prevalence of gout within families varies widely. However, approximately 25% of the relatives of gout patients will have hyperuricaemia.

Clinical manifestations

The classic mode of presentation is sudden intense inflammation of the *first metatarsophalangeal joint* often waking the patient in the middle of the night. The joint becomes acutely swollen and tender and the skin overlying it takes on a reddish-purple hue and often desquamates. The patient experiences excruciating pain and is unable to bear the weight of the bedclothes on the joint. Sometimes the patient is even unable to suffer the presence of other people in the same room for fear of jarring the inflamed joint.

◄ Acute gout attacks often occur at night and wake the patient

◄ The pain is excruciating with *marked* signs of inflammation.

Other joints such as the *knees, wrists* and *interphalangeal joints* can also be affected in the same patient (*polyarticular gout*). When this occurs diagnostic confusion can arise and conditions such as psoriatic arthritis and rheumatoid arthritis must be considered in the differential diagnosis. However, the suddenness and intensity of the attacks are really only paralleled by pseudogout (*see below*) and occasionally infective arthritis. Rarely, synovial joints in the spine including the sacro-iliac joints can be affected.

The acute attack usually settles in 5–10 days and some patients only experience one attack in their lifetime. Other patients suffer recurrent attacks, often in the same joint(s), and a previous history of similar attacks is helpful in making a clinical diagnosis. As the attacks increase in frequency then characteristic joint damage results. The attacks may be accompanied by *fever* and *rigors*.

Associated features

The tophus. In addition to the synovial membranes monosodium urate crystals may be deposited in any soft tissue in patients with hyperuricaemia. When this occurs extensive tissue destruction results and the lesion is known as a *tophus*. This comprises necrotic tissue and a massive collection of urate

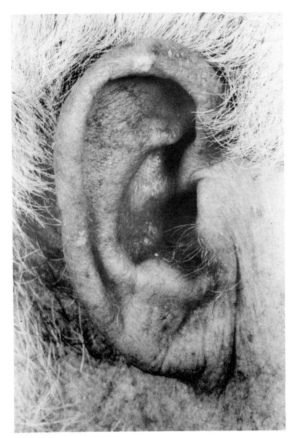

Fig. 8.5. Gouty tophus in the ear.

crystals often surrounded by a zone of calcification. Patients possessing these lesions are said to have *chronic tophaceous gout* whether or not they experience episodes of acute gouty arthritis — though most of them will. The common sites for tophi are:

◄ Not all patients with tophi suffer gouty arthritis.

1. The outer helix of the ear (*Fig.* 8.5)
2. In the skin overlying joints and tendons
3. In juxta-articular bone when they give rise to a typical radiological picture (*see Fig.* 8.4)
4. Kidney (*see below*)

A search for gouty tophi must be made in every patient with gouty arthritis as they indicate considerable tissue deposition of urate and are one of the indications for long-term treatment to lower the serum uric acid.

◄ The presence of tophi is an indication for long-term drug treatment.

Renal involvement. Sodium urate may be deposited in the renal parenchyma, particularly in the medulla where the pH of the environment is conducive to its precipitation. Marked renal damage and tophus formation may result (*gouty kidney*) and *hypertension* and *renal failure* occur as late sequelae. Fortunately, with modern, judicious drug treatment this complication is now rare. Urate stones can form giving rise to considerable distress and may be the presenting feature of hyperuricaemia. Massive tubular deposition of urate causing acute renal failure has been recorded in patients with myeloproliferative disorders treated with aggressive chemotherapy.

◀ Urolithiasis may be a presenting feature of hyperuricaemia.

Hypertension, coronary artery disease and hyperlipidaemia. All these conditions are associated with an increased incidence of gout and it is a wise precaution to screen all gouty patients for them after the initial diagnosis has been made. The exact inter-relationships between these conditions and gout are unknown and there is no direct evidence, for instance, that coronary artery disease is caused by a raised serum uric acid *per se* but in several population surveys the two conditions were seen in association. The association of gout with *Type 4 hyperbetalipoproteinaemia* is well documented.

Obesity. The association here is probably due to the fact that obese patients are more prone to ketoacidosis. This is particularly so during periods of severe dieting.

◀ Severe dieting in obese patients may precipitate gout.

Diabetes. Diabetes is also associated with gout — again probably due to the fact that diabetics are more prone to ketoacidosis.

Investigations

Crystal analysis. The only irrefutable laboratory evidence of gout is the identification of negatively birefringent crystals of monosodium urate in a sample of synovial fluid or material extruded from a tophus. All patients with an unexplained monoarthritis and a synovial effusion should have synovial fluid samples sent for polarizing microscopy. The synovial fluid in acute gout has a high polymorphonuclear leucocyte cell count in common with all acute inflammatory joint effusions.

◀ All patients with an unexplained monoarthritis should undergo crystal analysis of the synovial fluid.

Serum uric acid. This is usually elevated during an acute attack but not in every case and a normal value does not rule out the diagnosis. Conversely, not every patient with an acute arthritis and a raised serum uric acid has gout.

◀ Not every patient with acute arthritis and a raised serum urate has gout.

ESR. This is often considerably elevated during an acute attack.

Full blood count. A polymorphonuclear leuco-cytosis is usually present.

Radiology. Radiographs are of little value in the acute attack. In longstanding gout typical juxta-articular bony destruction comprising of punched-out lesions can be seen particularly in the first metatarsophalangeal joint (*see Fig.* 8.4). Calcifica-tion in and around these lesions is not uncommon.

Assessment of renal function (urea and electrolytes, serum and creatinine and MSU)
This is extremely important in all patients with gout. Renal impairment may be the cause of the hyperuricaemia and gout or the result of deposition of sodium urate in the renal parenchyma (*gouty nephropathy, see above*). Careful assessment of renal function in these patients is mandatory as it influences the course of treatment.

◀ Renal function should be assessed in all patients with gout.

Treatment
The aims of treatment are:
1. Pain relief during the acute attack
2. Prevention of further attacks
3. Treatment of associated disease, e.g. renal involvement, hypertension, hyperlipidaemia, obesity, etc.

Pain relief during an acute attack. Strong *anti-inflammatory drugs* are required to alleviate the excruciating pain of acute gout. Indomethacin in full dosage (50mg q.d.s.) is the traditional non-steroidal anti-inflammatory drug that is employed provided it can be tolerated by the patient. Other drugs in this group such as azapropazone may also be used. In addition to their anti-inflammatory effect, all these drugs increase the renal excretion of uric acid, i.e. are *uricosuric*. This effect is not very important therapeutically as it is fairly weak and short lived.

Aspirin-containing preparations are contraindicated for the reasons already described.

◀ Low-dose aspirin and aspirin-containing preparations may precipitate acute gout.

Colchicine a time-honoured treatment in gout, is still used for recalcitrant cases though it has become less favoured since the advent of the newer anti-inflammatory drugs. The initial dose is 0·5 mg q.d.s. or up to 2-hourly if required, reducing to 0·5 mg b.d. as the attack subsides. There is a high incidence of gastric irritation with this drug and diarrhoea is common. Its mode of action is not entirely understood but it is known to inhibit leucocyte migration to sites of inflammation and to stabilize lysosome membranes.

Corticosteroids, e.g. *prednisolone* (15 mg daily), are occasionally required but should only be used on a short-term basis. They may also be given by intra-articular injection.

Analgesics such as panadol and dihydrocodeine can be used as adjuncts to therapy during the acute phase.

Prevention of further attacks. Gout prophylaxis has become increasingly possible with the advent of the drug *allopurinol* which is a specific inhibitor of xanthine oxidase (*see Fig.* 8.1) and thereby reduces the serum uric acid.

◀ Allopurinol should not be used during or immediately after an acute attack.

Tophaceous deposits can also be reduced and sometimes disappear during treatment with this drug. It is contraindicated during an acute attack or during the phase immediately following an attack as it can exacerbate gout in these conditions. It is also given prophylactically in patients undergoing treatment for myeloproliferative disorders when the serum uric acid can rise to very high levels and result in renal damage (*see above*).

◀ Gout prophylaxis should be used in
• patients with recurrent attacks
• patients with tophaceous deposits
• gouty kidney.

Other agents, which work by increasing the renal excretion of uric acid (*uricosuric agents*), can also be used prophylactically. *Probenecid* (0·5–2 g per day) and *sulphinpyrazone* (50–400 mg daily) are both effective uricosuric agents. These drugs are contra-indicated in patients with renal damage, particularly those with a gouty kidney as they can exacerbate renal failure by increasing the likelihood of pre-cipitation of urate in the kidney. This tendency can be offset by alkalization of the urine to increase the solubility of urate but since the discovery of allopurinol the use of uricosuric agents is only necessary in a few patients when effective control cannot be achieved by the use of allopurinol alone. They are also useful in the small group of patients who can be proved to be under-excretors of uric acid. Colchicine at a dose of 0·5 mg t.d.s. has also been used as a prophylactic but its spectrum of side-effects, e.g. skin rashes, gastric intolerance, diarrhoea and rarely blood dyscrasias, tends to limit its use.

The place of *diet* in control of gout is somewhat controversial. The consensus is that it would seem sensible to advise patients to avoid food containing high concentrations of purines. Those whose alcohol intake is high should be advised to reduce this to more acceptable levels. In this respect it is pertinent to point out that there is a distinct '*gouty person-ality*'. Thus the typical patient is a middle-aged, hard working, jovial man leading a fairly stressful existence and with a proclivity for over-indulgence in the good life especially in terms of food and drink.

Treatment of hyperuricaemia
Treatment of hyperuricaemic patients without gouty arthritis should be limited to those whose serum uric acid levels are in excess of 9 mg% (0·54 mmol/l) or who have evidence of tophaceous deposits. Allopurinol is the drug of choice and treatment needs to be life-long. Patients with hyperuricaemic nephropathy should be treated vigorously and renal function monitored carefully. Fortunately this group of patients is becoming increasingly small as effective prophylaxis of hyperuricaemia has become possible.

◀ Hyperuricaemic patients only require treatment if:
- serum urate exceeds 0·54 mmol/l
- they have tophi
- there is evidence of 'gouty kidney', e.g. urolithiasis.

Treatment for associated disease
Obese gouty patients should be encouraged to diet, but crash diets are to be avoided as they induce lactic acidaemia which increases the risk of urate deposition. Patients with hyperlipidaemia are treated with low-fat diets in an attempt to mitigate the development of coronary artery disease.

Hypertension is treated in a standard manner, e.g. beta blockers, hydralazine, but the use of thiazide diuretics should be avoided as they can precipitate an attack.

Renal damage secondary to hyperuricaemia and tophaceous deposits is treated with allopurinol as previously indicated. Although this treatment halts the progress of further deposition of urate, renal function is usually already severely impaired and remains so.

Pseudogout and chondracalcinosis

Pseudogout is an acute synovitis resulting from the deposition of crystals of *calcium pyrophosphate* within joints. Clinically it resembles gout. It is associated with *chondrocalcinosis* which is a very common condition usually affecting ageing cartilage and results from calcium pyrophosphate deposition within the cartilage matrix, especially fibrocartilage. Calcium pyrophosphate is also deposited in the menisci and occasionally within ligaments. It can be detected radiologically (*Fig.* 8.6), and its presence is often associated with degenerative joint changes. Joints in which chondrocalcinosis can be most easily and most often identified are the *wrists, knees* and *pubic symphysis*.

◀ Chondrocalcinosis is most commonly identified in knees, wrists and pubic symphysis.

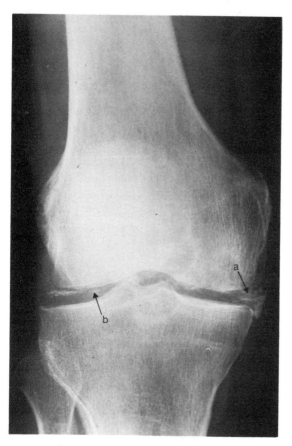

Fig. 8.6. Radiograph showing chondrocalcinosis in the knee joint. Calcium pyrophosphate deposited in: (*a*) the menisci; (*b*) the articular cartilage.

Aetiology

An acute attack of pseudogout is probably caused by shedding of calcium pyrophosphate crystals from the articular cartilage into the joint cavity where they can induce an intense inflammatory reaction. There is, however, no direct evidence for this mechanism and there may be other mechanisms whereby calcium pyrophosphate crystals precipitate in joints.

The causes of chondrocalcinosis are unknown. There is some evidence to suggest that calcium pyrophosphate, produced by chondrocytes, is deposited in the mucopolysaccharide matrix of the cartilage as calcium pyrophosphate crystals. Some authorities believe it to be a 'natural phenomenon' associated with ageing, and radiological prevalence of chondrocalcinosis increases with age as does osteoarthritis (*see* Chapter 2). In one survey of an elderly population (mean age 83 years) 26% had chondrocalcinosis.

Whether chondrocalcinosis is a causative factor in osteoarthritis is still hotly debated but certain diseases do have an interesting association with chondrocalcinosis, the most prominent in this respect being;

1. Hyperparathyroidism
2. Haemochromatosis
3. Diabetes
4. Ochronosis (alkaptonuria)
5. Wilson's disease

It is important to note that not all patients with chondrocalcinosis have attacks of pseudogout. The exact incidence of pseudogout in patients with chondrocalcinosis is unknown. It is highly likely that many cases go undetected because of inadequate synovial fluid analysis and some undoubtedly are misdiagnosed as gout.

◀ Not all patients with chondrocalcinosis develop pseudogout.

Clinical features

Pseudogout affects middle-aged and elderly patients — the male/female ratio being equal. The acute attack may be indistinguishable from gout, particularly when the first metatarsophalangeal joint is involved. Like gout, it usually presents as a mono-articular arthritis; the most common joint to be involved is the *knee* but the *shoulders* and *wrists* and indeed any synovial joint can be affected.

◀ Attacks of pseudogout are clinically indistinguishable from those of gout.

◀ Pseudogout attacks are most common in the knee.

The common presentation is in a patient with known osteoarthritis who suddenly develops an acute synovitis in one knee. The differential diagnosis is between gout, pseudogout and infective arthritis. Synovial fluid aspiration with crystal analysis is mandatory. The attacks are self-limiting and occasionally occur in 'clusters' over a short period of time leaving long symptom-free intervals. Like gout attacks they can be precipitated by:
1. *Surgery*
2. *Acute medical episodes* – such as *strokes* and *myocardial infarction*, or by
3. *Trauma*

Investigations

Synovial fluid analysis. During an attack this will reveal inflammatory fluid of low viscosity and high polymorpholeucocyte count. Under the polarizing microscope weakly positive birefringent crystals of calcium pyrophosphate will be seen. Polarizing microscopy is the only certain way of making a diagnosis in this condition. Synovial fluid culture is negative.

ESR. This is often elevated in the acute attack.

Full blood count. There is occasionally a mild polymorpholeucocytosis.

Radiology. Chondrocalcinosis is most easily seen in the wrists, knees and pubic symphysis.

Treatment

Chondrocalcinosis itself needs no treatment. Acute pseudogout is treated with *non-steroidal anti-inflammatory* drugs such as indomethacin and azapropazone. Occasionally *intra-articular steroids* are required and are very effective. The majority of patients will also be suffering from osteoarthritis. Standard treatment regimes are used in these cases (*see* Chapter 2) including joint replacement when required.

Further Reading

Dieppe P. (1981) Crystal induced arthropathies and osteoarthritis. In: W. Watson Buchanan and W. Carson Dick (ed.) *Recent Advances in Rheumatology 2*. Edinburgh, Churchill Livingstone.

Wyngaarden J. B. and Kelley W. M. (1971) *Gout and Hyperuricaemia*. New York, Grune & Stratton.

Polymyalgia rheumatica

9

The clinical features of this very important condition were rediscovered and described in detail by Barber in 1957. Earlier descriptions, however, do exist in the literature, but the most useful definition was given by Healey, Parker and Wilske in 1971: 'Polymalgia rheumatica, a syndrome of older patients, is characterized by pain and stiffness of the shoulder, or pelvic girdle muscles, without weakness or atrophy. These symptoms persist for at least a month, with a sedimentation rate greater than 50 mm/h and dramatic relief of symptoms with the use of steroids.'

It is associated with an arteritis, characterized by the presence of *multinucleate giant cells* in the media of the affected vessels and known as *giant-cell arteritis*. Giant-cell arteritis gives rise to the most dangerous and hence the most important complication of polymyalgia rheumatica — *blindness*.

◄ The main clinical characteristics of PMR are:
- Pain and stiffness around shoulder and/or pelvic girdle
- Age group 50+ years
- High ESR
- Prompt symptomatic response to steroids.

◄ Giant-cell arteritis is the most dangerous complication of PMR and can cause blindness.

Aetiology and pathology
The aetiology of polymyalgia rheumatica (PMR) is unknown. It is much more common in women. An infective, possibly viral, aetiology may explain the curious seasonal variation in the incidence of PMR. Some patients may have a prodromal 'flu-like illness and an association with upper respiratory tract infections has been reported but as yet specific viral studies in PMR have proved negative. *Familial aggregation* of PMR has been reported suggesting a possible genetic influence. Why it should be a disease confined to the older generation (50+ years) is not understood.

◄ PMR is more common in females.

In those cases complicated by arteritis, arterial biopsy appearances are characteristic. Large and medium-sized arteries are usually affected and all layers of the arterial wall are involved, i.e. *panarteritis*. The histological features are:
1. Narrowing of the lumen due to intimal proliferation
2. Thrombosis (secondary)
3. Multinucleate giant cells and monocytic infiltration of the media
4. Fragmentation of the internal elastic lamina
5. Infiltration of the adventitia with chronic inflammatory cells and fibrous tissue

The arteries most commonly involved are the extracranial arteries, especially the temporal arteries and less commonly the occipital arteries. The retinal artery may be affected and cause the most feared complication of PMR, that of blindness (fortunately usually monocular). Rarely, intracranial arteries are affected leading to stroke and, infrequently, cortical blindness. It is unusual for the arteritis to spread beyond the head and neck.

Considering the severity of muscular symptoms, surprisingly little is found on histological examination of affected muscles. Occasionally there may be some non-specific muscle fibre atrophy.

◀ Muscle histology and enzymes are normal.

Clinical features

1. Muscle stiffness and pain. This is the most prominent feature of PMR. It may be sudden in onset and often the patient claims to have woken one morning with severe stiffness around the shoulders which gradually wears off as the day progresses. The muscle symptoms, however, may be more insidious and the patient may have suffered them for some considerable time before consulting the doctor. The shoulder girdle is the site of predilection, though pelvic girdle muscles (buttocks and thighs) may be involved when the patient complains of pain and stiffness on sitting. Muscle tenderness, particularly at the root of the neck and over the shoulders, sometimes occurs but profound tenderness and weakness such as occur in polymyositis are not features of PMR.

2. General malaise. Patients often feel generally unwell during the course of the disease. Weight loss and depression are not uncommon and sometimes precede the onset of myalgia; a low-grade pyrexia also occurs.

◄ Weight loss and depression may precede the onset of muscle symptoms.

3. Joint pain. A mild synovitis of the peripheral joints, particularly the wrists and shoulders, occurs but is not usually prominent. Joint symptoms and signs should always alert one to the possibility of late onset rheumatoid disease. PMR presenting as bilateral shoulder capsulitis in an elderly person is not uncommon. Swelling of the manubriosternal and sternoclavicular joints may occur.

◄ A mild synovitis occurs in PMR, but is never as severe as that seen in RA.

4. Arteritic symptoms. These can be extremely variable and comprise:
- Headache
- Tenderness over the temporal arteries, e.g. patient unable to wear a hat because of pain. The affected arteries may also be non-pulsatile.
- Cervical and occipital pain and tenderness due to occipital arteritis
- Visual disturbance, e.g. transient loss, blurring and occasionally sudden monocular blindness due to retinal arteritis. Diplopia and orbital pain may result from involvement of vessels supplying the extra-ocular musculature
- Neurological symptoms due to intracranial arteritis, e.g. hemiparesis, are rare
- Jaw claudication on mastication due to involvement of vessels supplying the masseter muscles

◄ Arteritis of the retinal artery leads to visual disturbance which may antedate the onset of sudden monocular blindness.

Investigations
ESR. This is elevated often to very high levels, sometimes in excess of 100mm/h. However, cases of active arteritis resulting in blindness have been reported in patients with normal ESR. A *persistently* normal ESR, however, only occurs in 1 or 2% of patients.

Plasma viscosity. As with the ESR, this is usually elevated but is normal in a minority of patients. Patients with both a normal plasma viscosity and ESR are extremely rare.

C-reactive protein (CRP). This protein is produced by the liver as 'an acute phase reactant'. It is elevated particularly in infections, inflammatory conditions, e.g. rheumatoid arthritis and ankylosing spondylitis, and also in malignancy. High levels of CRP may be encountered in PMR.

Full blood count. A normochromic, normocytic anaemia develops as the disease progresses.

Immunoglobulins. A non-specific rise in alpha-2 globulin is common and revealed on protein electrophoresis. There may also be a polyclonal rise in immunoglobulins.

Temporal artery biopsy. The place of temporal artery biopsy in the diagnosis of PMR and giant-cell arteritis is still the subject of much debate. Of those patients with myalgic symptoms alone 40% can be shown to have histological evidence of an arteritis on blind temporal artery biopsy. Conversely, in one series of 61 patients with biopsy-proven temporal arteritis, only 11 did not have symptoms of PMR. These statistics help to illustrate how closely arteritis and PMR are associated. The arteritis may be very patchy and a negative biopsy does not rule out an active arteritis. This fact obviously throws some doubt on biopsy as a reliable diagnostic tool. It is the authors' experience that temporal artery biopsy is not necessary for diagnosis and should never be a cause for delaying the institution of effective corticosteroid treatment (*see below*).

Muscle studies
- Muscle enzymes are normal
- Electromyographic studies show non-specific changes. Occasionally a myopathic pattern may be shown
- Muscle biopsy is essentially normal and not diagnostic

Liver function tests. Approximately 20% of patients can be shown to have elevated *alkaline phosphatase* levels during active phases of the disease.

Conditions which masquerade as PMR

1. Rheumatoid arthritis. Late onset rheumatoid disease may have a polymyalgic onset. Patients with joint symptoms, as well as myalgia, should always be followed closely and screened for rheumatoid disease.

2. Multiple myeloma and disseminated malignancy. Although there is no direct relationship between PMR and these conditions, they can give rise to myalgic symptoms and be associated with a raised ESR. Hence diagnostic confusion may arise.

3. Cervical spondylosis (*see* Chapter 4). This condition gives rise to cervical and shoulder girdle pain, often with early morning exacerbations. It is not, however, associated with a raised ESR or plasma viscosity. It is usually relieved by rest. Radiological evidence of cervical spondylosis is unhelpful, as in the older age group it is an invariable finding.

◄ Cervical spondylosis may give rise to similar symptoms to PMR but is not associated with a raised ESR.

Treatment
Once the diagnosis has been made treatment should be started immediately. In those patients with myalgic symptoms alone, prednisolone (enteric coated) should be given at a dose of 15 mg daily. If an arteritis is suspected, and particularly if visual symptoms are present, the dose should be 30–60 mg daily. This dose should be maintained until the ESR and symptoms are controlled and then the dose can be gradually reduced to a maintenance dose, usually between 7·5 and 15 mg. The dose should be titrated against the ESR but two notes of caution should be made here:

◄ Once the diagnosis of PMR has been made, treatment with corticosteroids should begin immediately.

1. Intercurrent infections may be the cause of a raised ESR and do not necessarily signify a relapse of the disease
2. A few patients maintain a normal ESR despite a relapse of their symptoms

Thus during follow-up a careful symptomatic history should be taken as well as blood tests for ESR and plasma viscosity.

Non-steroidal anti-inflammatory drugs, particularly indomethacin and high-dose salicylates, will control symptoms but not an underlying arteritis and therefore they are not to be recommended.

◄ NSAIDs may abolish the symptoms of PMR but do not prevent arteritis.

The response to corticosteroids is diagnostic and within 24 h the majority of patients will be symptom-free and claiming a miraculous cure.

◄ Response to corticosteroids is dramatic and within 24 h.

Prognosis
Untreated the disease is said to run a course of some 18 months to 2 years. Relapses are common.

◄ The disease normally runs a 2-year course but relapses are common.

The administration of steroids does not shorten the duration of the disease but diminishes greatly the chance of blindness. Of those patients with arteritis, some 40% will develop the visual symptoms, including blindness, at some stage of their disease unless they are treated with corticosteroids. Steroid dosage is gradually reduced after 18 months, treatment and then withdrawn completely provided there has been no relapse of symptoms or the ESR does not rise. Patients should be followed up for at least 6 months after withdrawal of steroids to ensure they are not going to suffer an early relapse.

Further Reading
Hazelman B. (1976) Giant cell arteritis and polymyalgia rheumatica. In: Hughes G.R.V. (ed.) *Modern Topics in Rheumatology*. London, Heinemann.

Paget's disease, osteomalacia and osteoporosis

Patients with these conditions not uncommonly present in the rheumatology clinic complaining of musculoskeletal pain and are thus important in rheumatological differential diagnosis.

Paget's disease (osteitis deformans)

Sir James Paget gave the first comprehensive review of this disease to the Medical and Chirurgical Society of London in 1876. The disease affects predominantly the over-50 age group and increases in incidence with age. It results in overgrowth, softening and deformity of bone, hence its other descriptive title *osteitis deformans*.

◀ Paget's disease is most common in the over-50 age group. It is slightly more common in men than women.

Prevalence, aetiology and pathology

The exact prevalence of Paget's disease is unknown as most cases remain asymptomatic and are often discovered on bone radiographs performed for other reasons. It is estimated that between 3 and 4% of the over-50 population in this country are affected by the disease, the figure rising to 9% in the 85+ age group. The disease shows a marked geographical variation, being rare in Africa, Japan and Scandinavia but common in the UK, USA and Australia. Racial differences are also apparent and a familial tendency has also been noted which suggests some genetic influence on the disease. Clustering of the disease in certain areas, most strikingly in the North Lancashire area of the UK, also suggests a genetic influence and/or infective aetiology. It is slightly more common in men than women.

◀ The majority of patients with Paget's disease are asymptomatic and are discovered incidentally on radiography. Pain is the most common presenting symptom.

152

Paget's disease predominantly affects the leg bones and the axial skeleton, including the skull. It is characterized by areas of excessive bone resorption (osteoclastic activity) and deposition (osteoblastic activity) and resultant disorganization of normal bony architecture. In addition, the vascularity of the bone is greatly increased. Radiologically these changes are seen as areas of lucency surrounded by dense sclerotic bone in which the normal trabecular pattern has been lost. The affected bones often expand in size, sometimes massively so (*Fig.* 10.1) and long bones bend and bow and bizarre deformities may occur.

◄ It predominantly affects the weight-bearing bones, the axial skeleton and the skull.

◄ Pagetic bone is highly vascular.

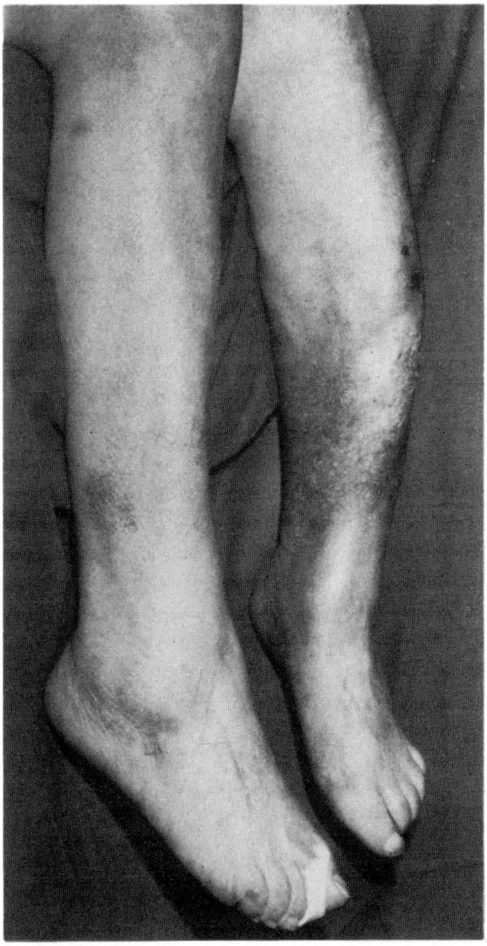

Fig. 10.1. Bowing of the tibia due to Paget's disease.

It is now thought that the primary defect in Paget's disease occurs in the osteoclasts which increase in both number and size in affected areas of bone. To compensate for the increase of osteoclastic activity, osteoblastic activity also increases. It is important to note that the normal 'coupling' of osteoclastic and osteoblastic activity remains but the rate of bone turn-over is grossly increased. Recently, large inclusion particles have been described in electron-micrographic sections of osteoclasts from involved bone giving rise to speculation that the cells have been infected with a slow virus. No particular virus has yet been identified but such a theory would be compatible with many of the known clinical and epidemiological features of the disease.

Clinical features

Bone pain is the most common symptom. The pain can be severe, is unrelieved by posture or rest, and may wake the patient at night. *Low back pain* and *hip pain* occur but may be due to coincidental degenerative joint disease. Limb deformity is often seen when the tibia is involved (*see Fig. 10.1*). Bowing of the tibia may lead to limb shortening and this predisposes to osteoarthritic changes in the contralateral leg, i.e. a long leg arthropathy (*see* Chapter 2).

In the *skull* the disease can cause frontal bossing and distorted facial features. Bony overgrowth may encroach upon the optic chiasma and the inner ear causing *blindness* and *deafness* respectively. Other cranial nerves may also become involved. Nerve and, occasionally, cordal entrapment may occur when the spine is affected.

◄ Involvement of the optic chiasma and inner ear may result in blindness and deafness respectively. Other cranial nerves may be involved if Paget's disease of the skull is severe.

A high cardiac output is common with a wide pulse pressure and collapsing pulse. This reflects the increased vascularity of involved bone and expansion of the peripheral vascular bed. Occasionally high output cardiac failure may supervene. The skin overlying affected bone may be warm and pink, as a result of increased vascularity.

◄ Increased vascularity of Pagetic bone results in a high cardiac output and occasionally cardiac failure.

A sudden increase in Pagetic bone pain may signify a *fracture* or malignant change. Fortunately, however, the development of *osteosarcoma* is very rare. It carries a poor prognosis.

◄ Sudden increase in bone pain may signify fracture or development of osteosarcoma.

Investigations

Radiology. The radiological appearances of Pagetic bone are diagnostic but extremely variable. Typically there is a mixture of changes seen within the bone:

1. Areas of resorption or osteolysis
2. Areas of thickened bone or osteosclerosis

The shape of the bone may be extremely distorted (*Fig.* 10.2). Sclerotic lesions in the vertebrae may mimic secondary deposits, e.g. from the prostate.

◄ Sclerotic lesions in vertebral bodies due to Paget's disease may mimic secondary deposits.

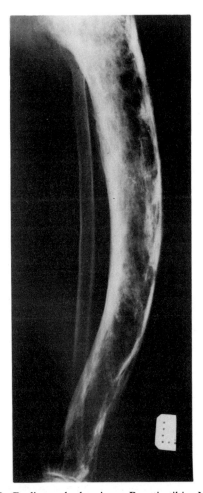

Fig. 10.2. Radiograph showing a Pagetic tibia. Note areas of lucency and sclerosis and bowing of bone.

Osteolytic lesions in the skull may not be accompanied by osteosclerosis and these lesions are known as *osteoporosis circumscripta*.

Laboratory investigations
1. The ESR may be elevated.
2. Biochemically, the increased rate of bone turnover is reflected in raised serum alkaline phosphatase (due to increased osteoblastic activity) and increased urinary hydroxyproline excretion (due to increased osteoclastic activity — the collagen matrix of bone is rich in hydroxyproline). Both these parameters can be used to monitor the activity of the disease.
3. Serum calcium and phosphate levels remain normal unless the patient undergoes a period of prolonged bed rest when serum calcium levels may become elevated.

Treatment
The main aim of treatment is to 'switch off' the increased bone turnover. This treatment can be directed against either the osteoclasts or the osteoblasts or both. Several drugs are now available that achieve this; some are too toxic in clinical use and only two are in general use at the present time. The indications for treatment are:
1. Bone pain
2. Before orthopaedic procedures on Pagetic bone, e.g. hip arthroplasty
3. To help heal fractures in Pagetic bone
4. Neurological complications, e.g. deafness, optic nerve damage

Note: Abnormal biochemistry itself is not an indication for treatment.

◀ Abnormal biochemistry, i.e. raised alkaline phosphatase, is not in itself an indication to treat Paget's disease.

1. Calcitonin. This is a peptide hormone secreted by the thyroid gland which inhibits osteoclastic activity. Several different preparations are now available — all are very expensive. The most widely used are salmon and porcine calcitonin. Both may produce allergic reactions. It is important that if major allergic reactions are to be avoided, a test dose is given subcutaneously before maintenance therapy begins. If no allergic response occurs after 24 h, then full dosage may be given. The dose ranges between 80 and 100 units twice weekly, though initially 100 units may be given daily to achieve more rapid control. Calcitonin usually gives satisfactory pain relief long before biochemical or radiological improvement in the disease occurs. In addition to its effect on osteoclasts, calcitonin is thought to exert an effect on bony vasculature and causes a decrease in blood flow through affected bone. Side-effects include diarrhoea, nausea, facial flushing and sweating.

2. Diphosphonates. These drugs are synthetic analogues of pyrophosphate — the main constituent of bone crystals. They act by stabilizing the bone crystals within the bony matrix and make them less vulnerable to osteoclastic resorption. They are active orally but are generally slower in their therapeutic effect than calcitonin. *Disodium etidronate* and *dichloromethylene diphosphonate* are both members of this group of drugs. The former and older drug has been more extensively used. It has been shown to have a favourable effect on the biochemistry and radiology of Paget's disease and is effective in relieving pain. Its major side-effect is that it can cause an increase in unmineralized osteoid, i.e. osteomalacia, if used in too high a dose. The recommended dose is 5 mg/kg/day for a 3–6-month course.

Other treatments
1. Non-steroidal anti-inflammatory drugs, particularly indomethacin and salicylates can be very effective in pain relief of Paget's disease.
2. Correction of any inequality of leg length by a suitable shoe-raise may help relieve pain and prevent further deterioration in secondary osteoarthritic joint changes.
3. Physiotherapy to encourage mobility and relieve concomitant osteoarthritic pain is of vital importance. Spinal supports are beneficial in some patients with vertebral Paget's disease.

◄ Side-effects of calcitonin are:
● diarrhoea
● nausea
● facial flushing and sweating

◄ Diphosphonates are synthetic analogues of pyrophosphate. Their main side-effect is to induce osteomalacia.

Osteomalacia
Vitamin D (cholecalciferol) is essential for the efficient formation of healthy bone. Deficiency of vitamin D results in abnormal osteoblastic activity and defective mineralization of the bony matrix (*osteoid*), i.e. osteomalacia. Vitamin D also enhances calcium absorption in the small bowel. It is derived from two sources:

1. The diet
2. By conversion of 7-dehydrocholesterol into vitamin D in the skin by the action of ultraviolet light
   It is hydroxylated in the liver and kidney to the active metabolite, 1,25-dihydroxyvitamin D. Certain individuals are particularly vulnerable to vitamin D deficiency, they are:

- The elderly (poor diet, lack of sunlight)
- Patients with malabsorption states
- Members of immigrant communities (dietary deficiency, reduced synthesis in pigmented skin)
- Renal failure (*renal rickets* due to defective hydroxylation into active metabolite)
- Children (increase in growing bone coupled with poor diet) — childhood osteomalacia, i.e. rickets.
- Pregnant and lactating women (increased demand)

◀ There are two sources of vitamin D:
- diet
- conversion of 7-dehydrocholesterol by UV light in the skin.

Clinical features

1. Bone pain. This may manifest itself as generalized musculoskeletal aching pains. It may be particularly prominent at the ends of long bones and simulate arthritic pain and generalized arthritis.

◀ Osteomalacia may cause bone pain which can be mistaken for a generalized arthritis.

2. Muscular weakness. This can at times be severe and be mistaken for a primary myopathy. Proximal muscles are affected most. Patients develop a waddling gait and have difficulty in rising from a chair.

3. Low back pain. This can masquerade as degenerative spinal disease but in the correct clinical setting and especially in a young patient, osteomalacia must be considered as a cause of low back pain.

4. Thoracic cage pain. This usually forms part of a more generalized skeletal pain. It is generally bilateral and tenderness may be elicited over the lower ribs.

Investigations

1. Radiology. In early disease bone radiographs may be entirely normal. As the disease becomes established the following features may be noted:
a. Increased lucency of bones (osteopenia)

b. Collapse of lumbar vertebrae
c. Looser zones (pseudofractures). These appear as lucent zones within otherwise normal bone. They are seen most frequently in the femoral neck, pubic bones, ribs and scapulae. They are due to uncalcified osteoid seams and are pathognomonic of osteomalacia. They can be painful
d. Bowing of weight-bearing long bones.
e. Gross bony distortion in children with rickets

◄ Looser zones, which are pathognomonic of osteomalacia, are most commonly seen in:
● femoral neck
● pubic bone
● ribs
● scapulae

2. *Laboratory investigations*
a. Haematologically there may be signs of malabsorption, e.g. low haemoglobin, macrocytosis.
b. Serum calcium is often normal (maintained by secondary hyperparathyroidism) but can be low. Alkaline phosphatase is usually high and serum phosphate is low.
c. Urinary calcium excretion is low.

3. *Bone biopsy.* This is rarely necessary but in the elderly, when osteoporosis and osteomalacia may coexist, it may be the only method of proving the diagnosis. Microscopically, large seams of uncalcified osteoid are seen.

◄ Bone biopsy in the elderly often reveals 'occult' osteomalacia as well as osteoporosis.

Treatment
This is achieved by the administration of vitamin D orally. Only occasionally is parenteral administration required. In malabsorption states and renal failure, large doses may be required but simple dietary deficiency can be corrected by small doses. Many foods are now fortified with vitamin D. Newer more potent metabolites of vitamin D are available, e.g. 1α-cholecalciferol, but these should be reserved for the more serious cases when a rapid response is required or when response to simple cholecalciferol is inadequate. When larger doses of vitamin D are being administered it is a wise precaution to check serum levels of calcium as hypercalcaemia may develop.

Osteoporosis
This condition results from the loss of bone substance. Calcification of osteoid is normal but there is a loss of the bony matrix. The bony

◄ Osteoporosis results from a loss of bone substance, including collagen fibre matrix.

trabeculae are thin and fewer in number and undergo microfractures and, as a result, the bone is weaker. This loss of bone is an inevitable consequence of ageing. Bone mass is maintained until early middle age (35–40) but thereafter bone mass slowly diminishes. This loss of bone varies greatly from individual to individual but is greatest in postmenopausal females and hence this group is more prone to osteoporosis than any other. Clinically relevant osteoporosis in males is rare. The causes of osteoporosis are:

◄ Postmenopausal females are most vulnerable to age-related osteoporosis.

1. Ageing — especially postmenopausal females
2. Disuse, e.g. arthritic conditions
3. Malabsorption states (osteoporosis usually seen in association with osteomalacia)
4. Cushing's syndrome
5. Iatrogenic Cushing's syndrome (administration of corticosteroids)
6. Thyrotoxicosis
7. Hyperparathyroidism
8. Multiple myeloma and occasionally other disseminated malignancies

Clinical features

Pain is not a feature of osteoporosis itself but results from bony fractures that eventually occur in the weakened bone. The commonest sites of fracture in long bones are the wrist (Colles' fracture) and the femoral neck. They often occur on minimal trauma. The vertebral bodies also undergo fracture and collapse (*Fig.* 10.3), and this results in spinal kyphosis and loss of height. The increase in mechanical stresses that this places on the spine causes a non-specific backache which is so characteristic of patients with osteoporosis. Occasionally a kyphosis can be so marked as to cause the ribs to impinge on the iliac crests causing considerable discomfort.

◄ Osteoporotic vertebral collapse results in a spinal kyphosis and loss of height. Back pain is a common presenting feature.

Investigations

1. Radiology. This is diagnostic but great care must be exercised in interpeting bone density on radiographs. Films of standard bones should be used for comparison and the radiological technique should be standardized as much as possible. Loss of bone

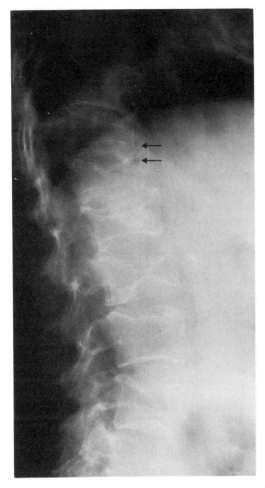

Fig. 10.3. Radiograph showing osteoporosis of the spine. Note increased lucency of bone and vertebral collapse (arrowed).

density is the most common sign of osteoporosis but other signs are also useful, particularly in the spine:
a. Wedge collapse (fracture) of vertebral bodies. It should be noted that a crushed vertebra has *increased* radiodensity.
b. Density of vertebral bodies closely approximates to that of the intervertebral discs and surrounding soft tissues.
c. Apparent increase in density of vertebral end-plates.

2. Biochemistry. This is unhelpful. Serum calcium and phosphate levels remain normal. Serum alkaline phosphatase is also normal unless recent fracture has occurred or there is coexisting osteomalacia or possible malignant disease.

Treatment

No single effective treatment as yet exists for osteoporosis but certain remedies at least hold some promise of ameliorating symptoms..

1. Physiotherapy and encouraging mobility. If bone is not stressed it becomes porotic, i.e. disuse atrophy, and this will occur regardless of the age of the patient. One of the most potent factors in maintaining bone mass is therefore exercise. It is vital that osteoporotic patients are encouraged to be as active as possible. This is best achieved by supervised physiotherapy and a regular daily exercise programme.

◀ One of the most potent methods of maintaining bone mass is exercise.

2. Analgesia. This is an important aspect of treatment and if successful it allows the patient to exercise more freely. Simple analgesics should be used and as the majority of patients are elderly and have compromised renal function, caution should be exercised in the prescription of analgesic drugs.

3. Calcium and vitamin D supplementation. If given early enough and long enough, there is some evidence to show that calcium supplementation to the diet may slow down the progress of osteoporosis. Many elderly patients also have concomitant osteomalacia (*see above*) and vitamin D supplementation will be required in these patients (the dual diagnosis being established by bone biopsy).

4. Anabolic steroids. These are sometimes given in conjunction with calcium supplements but there is no firm evidence of their efficacy in osteoporosis. In addition they do have side-effects, e.g. hirsutism, cholestatic jaundice, etc.

5. Oestrogen therapy. The place of oestrogen therapy in osteoporosis is still somewhat controversial. There is, however, definite evidence that oestrogens will reverse the osteoporosis that occurs in oophorectomized females and also in postmenopausal females. To be effective it has to be given early and prophylactically. However, side-effects òf long-term oestrogen therapy, e.g. thromboembolic disease, postmenopausal bleeding and possibly an increased incidence of uterine cancer, are such that it has not yet come into general use.

Further Reading
Hamby R. C. (1981) *Paget's Disease of Bone*. Endocrinology and Metabolism Series. Vol. 1. New York, Praeger.

Infective arthritis   11

Infective arthritis, fortunately, is rare but still clinically important despite the widespread use of modern antibiotics. Failure to recognize it and treat accordingly results in considerable morbidity and even mortality. Normal joints in healthy people are seldom infected except when the joint space is penetrated by a foreign body, e.g. nail, rose thorn, etc. However, many predisposing factors exist which make joints more vulnerable to infection and these are listed in *Table 11.1*.

◀ Normal joints seldom become infected.

Clinical features
- Swinging pyrexia
- Rigors
- General debility

These are often associated features of infective arthritis though they are not invariable.

Peripheral joints

Joint pain is usually severe and signs of inflammation (effusion, heat and redness) intense. Onset of the *loss of function* is rapid and both active and passive movement of the joint is steadfastly resisted by the patient. Exceptions to these general rules may occur in rheumatoid patients who are also taking steroids when infection of a joint(s) can be very insidious with few physical findings. The picture is further complicated by the fact that rheumatoid synovitis can coexist and differentiating infection from it is often impossible unless synovial fluid is sent for culture. In the majority of cases, *haematogenous*

◀ Movements of infected joints are severely limited.

◀ Joint infection in RA may be insidious especially in those patients taking steroids. They may also be misdiagnosed as rheumatoid synovitis.

Table 11.1.   Predisposing factors in joint infection

1. Previous joint damage
      Rheumatoid arthritis
      Osteoarthritis
      Other destructive arthropathy

2. General debility and systemic disease (often resulting in disordered neutrophil and/or B-cell function)
      Rheumatoid arthritis
      The elderly and neonates
      Alcoholics
      Uraemia
      Malignancy
      Myeloproliferative disorders
      Diabetes
      SLE

3. Iatrogenic immunosuppression
      Corticosteroids
      Cytotoxic and immunosuppressive drugs

4. Sickle-cell disease (more commonly predisposes to osteomyelitis that may secondarily involve joints)

5. Drug abusers (intravenous)

6. Coexisting infection elsewhere
      Staphylococcal abscesses
      Pulmonary tuberculosis. Bronchiectasis
      Enteric fever (more commonly causes reactive arthritis, *see* Chapter 7)
7. Orthopaedic procedures (especially arthroplasty)

spread from some primary focus is responsible, e.g. *skin infection, urinary tract infection, bronchiectasis*, and these should be diligently sought as they will give vital clues as to the nature of the possible causative organisms (*Table* 11.2).

Table 11.2.   The more common organisms encountered in joint infections

1. Staphylococci (commonest)
2. Streptococci (including pneumococci)
3. *Haemophilus influenzae* (especially in children)
4. *Escherichia coli*, pseudomonas
5. *Neisseria gonorrhoeae*
6. *Neisseria meningitidis* (meningococci) (especially in children)
7. Salmonellae (children, large joints). Also salmonella in sickle-cell anaemia
8. *Mycobacterium tuberculosis*

Infections of the spine (including the sacro-iliac joints) These are usually more difficult to diagnose and often only when radiological damage is observed is the true cause of symptoms revealed. Non-specific backache in association with pyrexia and general debility (especially weight loss) should always arouse suspicion and predisposing factors should be sought. *Tuberculosis* still remains the most common infection of the spine, though *staphylococcal* and *gram-negative* infections also occur. *Brucellosis* also has a curious predilection for the spine and sacro-iliac joints.

◄ Infections of the spine may go undiagnosed until radiological damage has occurred.

Investigations

Arthrocentesis
Aspiration of joint fluid for microscopy and culture is the single most important investigation in the diagnosis of joint infections. The rule is: if in doubt about the cause of an effusion, aspirate and culture. Characteristics of infected fluid are:
- Thin
- Cloudy
- Sometimes bloodstained
- High polymorphonuclear count (greater than 50,000/mm^3)
- Simple gram stain will be positive in over 50% of cases

◄ Aspiration and culture of synovial fluid is mandatory if there is a clinical suspicion of infective arthritis. Blood cultures should be taken simultaneously.

Blood cultures
Blood samples should always be taken at the time of arthrocentesis.

Blood glucose and synovial fluid glucose
Synovial fluid glucose is usually low in joint infections when compared with blood glucose. This finding, however, is somewhat variable, e.g. non-infected rheumatoid synovial fluid often has a low glucose content, tuberculous fluid may have a normal glucose content.

Full blood count and ESR
ESR is elevated. A neutrophilia is common.

Radiographs
These are of little value in acute joint infections showing only soft-tissue swelling. In more chronic

cases *juxta-articular osteoporosis* occurs and *loss of cartilage* is evidenced by narrowing of the joint space. Bony changes due to osteomyelitis are a late manifestation, though in the spine may be the first direct evidence of infection. In the spine the disc is often the seat of infection and *discitis*, seen as sclerosis of surrounding vertebral bone and eventually disc destruction, is usually the first sign.

Gonococcal arthritis

The prevalence of gonococcal infection has increased markedly over the past decade. Gonococcal arthritis has become the most common form of infective arthritis in the USA. The number of cases occurring in this country in young sexually active people is also increasing. It is more common in females than males. Symptoms from the primary site of infection, e.g. genitalia, rectum or pharynx, may be minimal and often the first presenting symptom of disseminated gonococcal infection is a *migratory polyarthritis* which usually localizes to a few joints, particularly the knees and ankles. Such a presentation in a young female should always arouse suspicion of a gonococcal infection. There may be a low-grade fever, rigors and a feeling of general malaise. A *tenosynovitis* may occur in conjunction with the arthritis, particularly affecting the extensor tendons of the hands and wrists.

◀ A migratory polyarthritis localizing to a few joints in a young female should always arouse suspicion of gonococcal infection.

The characteristic *rash*, comprising sparsely scattered vesicular, pustular lesions occurring mainly on the extremities, is common. A more transient maculopapular rash occurs less frequently.

Investigations

1. Full blood count; neutrophilia is common.
2. Blood cultures. Occasionally *Neisseria gonorrhoeae* can be cultured from the blood during the bacteriaemic stages of the disease when culture of swabs taken from the sites of infection have been negative.
3. *Synovial fluid analysis*. As in other forms of infective arthritis, this investigation is mandatory. The fluid has a high neutrophil count and is typically inflammatory in appearance. Gram stain may reveal gonococci as *gram-negative intracellular diplococci*,

but even if identified, culture of synovial fluid may be negative owing to the fastidious culture requirements of the organism.

◀ Culture of synovial fluid may be negative in gonococcal arthritis.

Tuberculous arthritis

This continues to be a clinical problem despite the dramatic fall in the prevalence of pulmonary tuberculosis over the past 20 years. It is becoming increasingly a problem of more elderly patients whereas it used to be more common in young adults. Other patients who are at risk are:

- The iatragenically immunosuppressed, e.g. those patients on cancer chemotherapy regimes
- Rheumatoid arthritics
- Rheumatoid and SLE patients on steroids
- The immigrant population, especially Asian

Clinical features

Onset is invariably insidious and pain is minimal. The usual signs of inflammation are absent and often the only abnormality is an effusion. Occasionally there may be *night sweats* and *rigors* which indicate transient bacteriaemia. A slowly progressive debility with weight loss is often present, however. Infection of tendon sheaths leading to *tenosynovitis* is now very rare.

◀ The onset of tuberculous arthritis is insidious and the usual signs of acute inflammation are often absent though an effusion is usually detectable. The spine is a common site of involvement.
◀ Joint signs in tuberculous arthritis may be limited to an effusion without signs of acute inflammation.

Investigations

These, too, are often unhelpful:
1. The Mantoux test may be negative.
2. A low-grade neutrophilia may be present. If the infection becomes chronic, a normochromic, normocytic anaemia develops.
3. The ESR is invariably elevated.
4. Synovial fluid is usually purulent but occasionally only a few pus cells are present. Routine microscopy for acid-fast bacilli is often negative and even specialized culture may be negative. Synovial biopsy, or synovectomy, is diagnostically much more

◀ Mantoux test may be negative.

reliable, often revealing typical cavitating granulomas around which acid-fast bacilli may be identified. Culture of such material is more likely to be positive than culture of synovial fluid.

◄ Culture of a synovial tissue biopsy is more likely to be positive than culture of synovial fluid.

Radiology. The most striking radiological feature of tuberculous arthritis is the involvement of the juxta-articular bone. Subchondral cysts are common and loss of bone may be severe ('disappearing joint syndrome'). The surrounding bone is very sclerotic. In early infections the radiological appearance is entirely non-specific consisting of soft-tissue swelling and juxta-articular osteoporosis.

Involvement of the spine (*Pott's disease*) is seen as a loss of disc height, sclerosis and erosion of the adjacent vertebral body and eventual collapse and formation of *gibbus* (hunch-back).

Treatment

Standard antituberculous treatment should be given as soon as the diagnosis is suspected. This usually comprises *rifampicin, isoniazid* and *ethambutol.* The former two drugs can be given in combination capsules (rimactazid). Treatment should be continued for at least 9 months. If response is satisfactory ethambutol may be discontinued after 3 months. In some patients in whom acid-fast bacilli cannot be identified microscopically, chemotherapy has to be given as a therapeutic trial as culture of tubercle takes a considerable time and may be negative. These patients should be followed up closely and monitored for a positive response to treatment, e.g. resolution of joint effusion, fall in ESR, improvement in radiological signs.

◄ Chemotherapy occasionally has to be given as a therapeutic trial in patients with tuberculous arthritis in whom tubercle bacilli have not been isolated but where there is a strong clinical suspicion of acid-fast infection.

Synovectomy of peripheral joints, particularly the knee and hip, is indicated in some patients under the cover of adequate chemotherapy .

Treatment of infective arthritis

1. Early diagnosis, which requires a high index of clinical suspicion and culture of synovial fluid, is vital in infective arthritis if irreversible cartilage damage is not to ensue.

2. Rest and control of pain are important aspects of treatment.

3. More important is the choice of antibiotic and its prompt administration at the right dose.

4. Surgical drainage of joints, particularly the hips, may be indicated and should be resorted to earlier rather than later, i.e. when there is insufficient response to conservative measures after 48h of treatment.

5. Repeated aspiration of joints as synovial fluid reaccumulates is often advocated but, in many cases this is extremely difficult as loculation of fluid occurs and for this reason formal surgical drainage is to be preferred.

◄ Early diagnosis which includes culture of synovial fluid is vital in the treatment of infective arthritis.

◄ Surgical drainage of involved joints should be performed early if there has not been a satisfactory response to antibiotics.

Choice of antibiotics

Often antibiotic therapy has to be given 'blind' and modified when the antibiotic sensitivities of the infecting organisms become known. The gram stain is very helpful in making a rational choice of antibiotic as indicated in *Table* 11.3. If there is a likely clinical source of infection, e.g. furuncle (*Staph. aureus*), urinary tract infection (gram-negative organisms), chest infections (pneumococci, haemophilus), then this also helps to rationalize the choice of antibiotic.

◄ The appearance of the gram film allows a more rational choice of antibiotic to be made in infective arthritis.

Method of administration of antibiotics

It is general practice to administer antibiotics *parenterally* (preferably intravenously) to ensure adequate tissue levels and penetration into purulent

Table 11.3. Gram stain and choice of antibiotics

Gram stain	Likely organism	Antibiotic
Gm +ve cocci	Staphylococcus (aureus)	Penicillinase stable penicillin e.g. flucloxacillin
	Streptococcus (pneumoniae, faecalis)	Penicillin G/V
Gm −ve cocci	N. gonorrhoeae	Penicillin G/ampicillin
Gm −ve bacilli	Haemophilus influenzae (children)	Ampicillin
	E. coli Pseudomonas Proteus	Aminoglycoside, cephalosporin

synovial fluid. Intra-articular antibiotics are not indicated. Once the infection is under control, the antibiotic should be continued orally with the exception of aminoglycosides which have to be given intramuscularly. In the case of staphylococcal infections, antibiotics should be continued for at least 3 months.

General measures
Rest in the initial stages helps speed recovery. Splintage of joints is rarely necessary and great care has to be taken to ensure that joints do not become stiffened or suffer contractures. To this end passive movements, supervised by a physiotherapist, are allowed in the acute stage and early mobilization achieved as the infection subsides to ensure that muscle wasting (particularly if the hip or knee is involved) is kept to a minimum.

◄ Passive and active physiotherapy are essential to prevent muscle wasting and joint contracture.

Viral arthritis
A number of viruses may cause an acute polyarthritis. The most common is rubella but others such as *mumps, infectious mononucleosis, hepatitis B* and *chickenpox* may be complicated by an acute self-limiting arthritis. They often occur in young people and the chief differential diagnosis, therefore, is rheumatoid arthritis and at presentation viral arthritis may be indistinguishable from acute rheumatoid disease.

◄ Viral polyarthritis may mimic acute rheumatoid arthritis.

Rubella arthritis
An acute polyarthritis may occur as a complication of a rubella infection. It usually follows the acute prodroma of coryza, fever and malaise but can occur before, during, after or even in the absence of the rash. It is most common in young adult females. The wrists, fingers and knees are typically involved with swelling and stiffness which may be severe. The arthritis lasts for between 2 and 30 days and resolves without any residual joint damage.

Synovial fluid analysis shows the predominance of mononuclear cells and rubella virus has been isolated from affected joints.

Treatment
Treatment is purely symptomatic with non-steroidal anti-inflammatory drugs.

It has become increasingly recognized since the introduction of the rubella immunization programme that the live attenuated viral strain used in the vaccine may also cause rubella arthritis.

◄ Rubella immunization may cause rubella arthritis.

Infectious mononucleosis

A true arthritis is rare during an attack of glandular fever. It usually takes the form of a transient monoarthritis of the knee or ankle. *Arthralgia*, which may be severe, is a much more common feature. A false positive test for rheumatoid factor may occur.

◄ A false positive test for rheumatoid factor may occur in glandular fever.

Mumps

Mumps arthritis usually affects young adult males. It tends to be *monoarticular* or *pauciarticular* involving the elbow, ankle and, less commonly, the knees. It usually occurs towards the end of the second week of infection, but may occur later as the acute salivary gland swelling is settling.

Hepatitis B

An *acute symmetrical polyarthritis* is not an uncommon complication of this infection and can occur at any time during the illness. It is thought to be immune complex mediated and is associated with a vasculitis. Hepatitis B surface antigen has been isolated from the synovial fluid of affected patients. Resolution occurs spontaneously and without any residual joint damage.

Viral arthralgia and myalgia

Symptoms of arthralgia and myalgia are extremely common and when associated with a 'flu-like' illness are assumed to have a viral aetiology. Viruses which are commonly implicated are: influenza, coxsackie and echo. Occasionally viral infections are complicated by erythema nodosum and a flitting arthritis is common in these cases.

Childhood arthritis   **12**

In this chapter we will deal with a variety of arthritides that affect children, i.e. any individual below the age of 16. The classification of childhood arthritis has undergone considerable rationalization in the past decade. Careful clinical research has led to an understanding that several different types of chronic arthritis are seen in childhood each with its own prognosis and spectrum of disease associations.

Musculoskeletal pain is a common symptom in children. In very young children it is often difficult and sometimes impossible to localize the pain to a particular joint or muscle group. For example, the complaint of 'all my leg hurts' is often made when examination reveals pathology clearly localized to the hip, knee or ankle. The child may be brought to the clinic by his parents who have noticed that he is *limping*. Careful history taking in the presence of a competent parent and meticulous clinical examination are especially relevant in this age group.

◀ Childhood arthritis may often present as a 'limp'.

The types of arthritis that affect children are listed in *Table* 12.1.

Infective and postviral arthritis
These conditions are discussed in Chapter 11.

Rheumatic fever
Rheumatic fever is a disease characterized by:
- Group A beta-haemolytic streptococcal infection (usually of the pharynx)
- Fever

Table 12.1.   Classification of childhood arthritis

Infective
   (or associated with infection)
      Bacterial
      Postviral (esp. rubella)
      Rheumatic fever
      Henoch–Schönlein purpura

Juvenile Chronic Arthritis
      Systemic juvenile chronic arthritis
         (Still's disease)
      Pauciarticular arthritis
      Seronegative polyarthritis
      Juvenile rheumatoid arthritis

Associated with other disease
      Psoriatic arthritis
      Inflammatory bowel disease
      Blood dyscrasias (esp. leukaemias)
      Collagen disease
         SLE
         PAN
         Dermatomyositis
         Scleroderma

Non-specific Articular and Periarticular Pain
'Orthopaedic' Conditions ('growing pains')
      Perthes' disease; Osgood–Schlatter's disease
      Slipped femoral epiphysis; Congenital dislocation
         of hip
      Epiphyseal dysplasia
      Scheuermann's disease, etc.

- Migratory polyarthritis
- Erythema marginatum
- Chorea
- Subcutaneous nodules

Males and females are equally affected, usually
between the ages of 5 and 15. It occurs rarely in
adults. Any individual may undergo several attacks.

◀ Rheumatic fever may
occur in adults.

Aetiology
Rheumatic fever and its sequelae are thought to be
the result of a heightened and abnormal tissue
response to infection by group A beta-haemolytic
streptococci. The evidence for streptococci being a
causative factor in the disease is epidemiological and
immunological. Group A beta-haemolytic streptococcal infections show a seasonal, climatic and social
class variation mirrored by rheumatic fever. Thus

there is an increased incidence in the autumn and winter, in social classes 4 and 5 and also in temperate climates. It is also well known that rheumatic fever occurs in epidemics associated with outbreaks of group A beta-haemolytic streptococcal infections, particularly in close-knit communities such as schools, prisons and army barracks. There is also a familial aggregation of the disease suggesting an infective aetiology.

◀ Rheumatic fever is more common in the autumn and winter and in social classes 4 and 5.

One of the most remarkable features of rheumatic fever is its declining incidence in 'high technology' communities. Like most infective diseases the advent of proper sanitation, civilized housing conditions and better nutrition have all helped towards eradicating the disease. It is also thought that the beta-haemolytic streptococcus may have altered its characteristics and become less virulent and less likely to trigger attacks of rheumatic fever in predisposed individuals.

The latent period between infection and manifestations of the disease has led to speculation that immunological mechanisms are operating in the pathogenesis of the disease. High titres of anti-streptococcal antibodies are usually found in patients with rheumatic fever and if taken early enough, pharyngeal swabs often reveal the presence of beta-haemolytic streptococci in the throat. This in itself is not proof that the organism is responsible for the disease as many individuals are *asymptomatic carriers*, but high and rising titres of anti-streptococcal antibodies are evidence of a pathologically significant infection. Not all individuals with beta-haemolytic streptococcal sore throats, however, develop the disease. There are thought to be two reasons for this:

1. There are many different types of streptococci and there is probably antigenic variation even within the Lancefield groups.
2. The host response to the infection is also variable and it may be that only certain genetically predisposed individuals will develop the disease following an infection with a specific type of streptococcus.

Rheumatic carditis, the most important complication of rheumatic fever, is thought to arise as a result of tissue damage caused by beta-haemolytic streptococcal antibodies that cross-react with cardiac

◀ Rheumatic carditis is the most important complication of rheumatic fever.

Table 12.2. Clinical features of rheumatic fever

- Sustained fever
- Flitting (migratory) polyarthritis
- Carditis
- Erythema marginatum
- Sydenham's chorea
- Subcutaneous nodules

muscle. The inference is that certain strains of beta-haemolytic streptococci share an antigenic determinant with cardiac tissue.

Clinical features
These are summarized in *Table* 12.2. Patients usually develop symptoms 1–2 weeks after a beta-haemolytic streptococcal throat infection. In some patients the throat infection may be asymptomatic. Onset is usually sudden and heralded by a *sustained fever*, general lethargy and joint pain.

◀ The fever of rheumatic fever is sustained.

Arthritis
This follows a very characteristic pattern — it is a *migratory polyarthritis* affecting large joints, e.g. wrists, elbows, knees and ankles and usually sparing the small joints of the hand and feet. A particular joint may only show evidence of inflammatory synovitis for 48h or less and then settle completely to be followed by a flare-up in another joint. Effusions are usually not large but synovial fluid is typically inflammatory in its characteristics (thin, turbid with a high polymorph count). The arthritis leaves no residual cartilage damage. A rare syndrome, first described by *Jaccoud*, is seen after repeated and severe attacks of rheumatic fever. Patients develop contractures of the flexor tendons and subluxation of the metocarpophalangeal joints with ulnar deviation. These deformities are passively correctable and painless. Similar deformities have been described in SLE (*see* Chapter 6).

◀ The arthritis characteristically 'flits' from joint to joint.

◀ Jaccoud's 'arthritis' is a rare chronic sequela of rheumatic fever.

Carditis
This is the most important complication of rheumatic fever which can lead to permanent tissue damage in and around the heart resulting in varying degrees of cardiac disability in later life. As the prevalence of rheumatic fever falls so does the prevalence of

rheumatic heart disease. All layers of the heart can be affected.

Pericarditis. Pericarditis presents with precordial chest pain, which is positional and worse on respiration. It can be associated with a pericardial effusion and cardiac constriction resulting in signs of right-sided cardiac failure.

Myocarditis. Myocarditis is indicated by a persistent tachycardia, present even after the fever has settled. Both these complications are accompanied by characteristic ECG changes, chief of which are a prolongation of the PR interval and/or QT interval, elevation of the ST segment and a variety of arrhythmias.

◄ Myocarditis is indicated by a persistent tachycardia and ECG changes.

Endocarditis. This is responsible for valvular deformity leading to stenosis or incompetence predominantly of the mitral valve, but the aortic valve and occasionally both valves may be involved. Only very rarely is the right side of the heart affected probably because the pressure gradients across the valves are less than they are on the left side of the heart. The earliest cardiac murmur to be heard in acute rheumatic fever is the *Carey Coombs murmur* which is a *mid-diastolic* bruit thought to be due to dilatation of the left ventricle. It often disappears without any sequelae but is sometimes followed by a rough low-pitched mid-diastolic murmur of *mitral stenosis* — indicative of permanent mitral valve damage secondary to inflammatory fibrosis of the valve cusps and chordae tendineae and constriction of the mitral valve ring. Congestive cardiac failure may develop in later life as a result of mitral stenosis and is often accompanied by *mitral incompetence* and not infrequently by atrial fibrillation. The risks of permanent valvular damage are increased if the patient suffers repeated attacks of rheumatic fever.

◄ Endocarditis results in deformity of the mitral and/or aortic valves.

◄ Risk of valvular damage is increased during repeated attacks of rheumatic fever.

Subcutaneous nodules
These occur in 'crops' over bony prominences, joints and tendons. They are usually measured in millimetres and can be tender and vary rapidly in size during the course of acute rheumatic fever. They thus differ from rheumatoid nodules clinically but histologically the differentiation is less clear (*see* Chapter 5). They comprise an outer layer of mononuclear cells classically arranged in a palisade

◄ Rheumatic nodules are small and non-tender and occur in 'crops'.

around a central area of necrosis and fibrosis. Occasional giant cells may be seen within the palisade. They disappear without any sequelae as the acute attack settles. Similar nodules can be seen in any layer of the heart when they are known as *Aschoff nodes.*

Erythema marginatum. Only about 5% of patients develop this characteristic rash. It occurs during the acute phases of the disease and comprises a macular rash with areas of central pallor surrounded by a red serpiginous border. Lesions are said to resemble a coastline map and are found mainly on the trunk. It can rarely occur in other conditions such as SLE and as a reaction to certain drugs.

Sydenham's chorea. This is the least common feature of rheumatic fever and it can occur in the absence of the characteristic arthritis. It is caused by a generalized *meningoencephalitis* and manifests itself as purposeless, writhing movements of the limbs and often emotional lability. Paralysis of the limb can ensue but this is rare and most cases are mild with occasional jerky movements of the limbs and a certain clumsiness. It is usually short-lived and recovery is complete.

Other associations such as *peritonitis* and *acute post-streptococcal glomerulonephritis* may occur.

Laboratory investigations
There is no diagnostic test for rheumatic fever. A throat swab will often reveal the presence of beta-haemolytic streptococci but this is by no means diagnostic for reasons already outlined.

ASO titres
A rising titre of antibodies to streptolysin O (a haemolysin produced by beta-haemolytic strepto-cocci) is indicative of recent beta-haemolytic strepto-coccal infection but is not a diagnostic test.

Rheumatoid factor
This is always negative. Patients with post-rheumatic chronic valvular heart disease may develop subacute bacterial endocarditis, a condition which is often associated with very high serum levels of rheumatoid factor (*see* Chapter 5).

◀ Patients with rheumatic valvular heart disease are at risk from subacute bacterial endocarditis.

ESR
This is always elevated, often to high levels.

Full blood count
A leucocytosis and normochromic, normocytic anaemia are common.

Radiology
Chest radiography is valuable in assessing cases with cardiac involvement, particularly in patients with pericarditis. More sophisticated techniques such as echocardiography are also invaluable in assessing pericardial effusions and valvular lesions. Joint radiographs are normal apart from showing non-specific soft-tissue swelling in affected joints.

Treatment
Bed rest and *salicylates* still remain the standard treatment for acute rheumatic fever. Aspirin should be given in the maximum tolerated dose (up to 100 mg/kg body weight). Inflamed joints should be rested but intermittently put through a passive range of movements by a physiotherapist. It is customary once the diagnosis has been made to administer *penicillin* in order to eradicate any remaining beta-haemolytic streptococcal infection. A 2-week course of penicillin G 250 mg q.d.s. is usually prescribed. Obligatory prophylaxis against subsequent attacks of rheumatic fever (during which irreversible cardiac damage is much more likely) is carried out usually for 5–10 years after the first attack or until the child leaves school and is given in the form of penicillin V 250 mg b.d. (it may also be given as monthly injections of the long-acting intramuscular benzathine penicillin 1 megaunit). In addition, extra antibiotic cover should be given during intercurrent infections and any elective surgical procedure, particularly *dental procedures*. In patients with rheumatic valvular heart disease, antibiotic cover should be given prophylactically during any surgical procedure that is embarked upon during their life as the risks of developing subacute bacterial endocarditis are high. In severe acute carditis usually accompanied by congestive cardiac failure, *steroids* have been said to reduce the severity of subsequent cardiac damage.

◄ Bed rest and salicylates are still the mainstay of treatment of rheumatic fever.

◄ Patients with valvular heart disease should have antibiotic cover during any surgical procedure.

Henoch–Schönlein purpura

This is an uncommon disease with a peak age of onset between 2 and 5 years though it has been recorded in adults. The cause is unknown but an association with streptococcal infection has been suggested. Pathologically it is a *generalized vasculitis* affecting:

- Skin
- Intestines
- Kidneys
- Rarely, the nervous system

The characteristic *purpuric rash* is seen on the lower legs, buttocks and arms. Lesions may coalesce to form large haemorrhagic spots. The patient feels ill and this is usually associated with *fever* and *leucocytosis*. Painful large joint *arthritis* is commonly seen with the rash. It can have a migratory quality but this is not usually as marked as it is with rheumatic fever. The arthritis settles without sequelae.

◀ The arthritis of Henoch–Schönlein purpura may have a migratory quality that settles without sequelae.

Abdominal pain may arise from two causes:
1. Intestinal bleeding which can be severe, and
2. Intussusception

both as a result of vasculitis and oedema of the intestinal wall. *Renal* involvement presenting as proteinuria and microscopic haematuria is seen in up to 70% of cases. An *acute glomerulonephritis* with renal failure is rare and severe renal involvement is usually confined to older children. *Meningeal* involvement results in *subarachnoid haemorrhages* and/or convulsions but these are rare complications.

Investigations

1. The ESR is elevated.
2. A leucocytosis is common. Platelet counts are normal and anaemia which can be of rapid onset occurs in those patients with gastrointestinal involvement.
3. Hess's test of capillary fragility is positive.
4. Examination of a midstream urine specimen is mandatory to detect renal involvement and also monitor progress of any renal lesion.

◀ Urine microscopy is vital in detecting early renal involvement.

5. The faeces should be examined for overt or occult intestinal haemorrhage.
6. Tests for rheumatoid factor are negative.

Treatment
Most cases settle spontaneously without sequelae. General supportive measures such as analgesia and non-steroidal anti-inflammatory drugs for joint pain should be given. Blood transfusion may be required for excessive bleeding. Intestinal intussusception sometimes settles spontaneously or may be reversed by a barium enema. Some patients require surgical correction.

Juvenile chronic arthritis
This is the term now in general use to describe a group of chronic arthritides that affect children. They differ from each other in their clinical expression, their prognosis and various laboratory and radiological parameters, but overlap between the various groups occurs frequently.

Systemic juvenile chronic arthritis
In 1897 George Frederick Still, whilst a medical registrar at the Hospital for Sick Children, Great Ormond Street, described a group of children with acute and chronic arthritis. He noted that 12 of the children with *acute arthritis* also had *lymphadeno-pathy*, *splenomegaly* and a *hectic fever*. This sub-group is now recognized as 'Still's disease' by many authorities although the eponym is often applied, somewhat misleadingly, to any child with chronic arthritis. Another feature of this group added since Still's classic description is an *evanescent rash*. The most common age of onset is under 5 but children of any age may be affected and even adult cases of the disease have now been described.

◀ Still's disease comprises acute arthritis, lymphadenopathy, splenomegaly and fever.

◀ Still's disease has been described in adults.

The *fever* is persistent and often lasts for days without an infective cause being identified. It is characteristically fluctuant and often returning to normal only to rise rapidly a few hours later. The *rash* appears during these febrile episodes and it, too, is intermittent disappearing in a matter of hours only to reappear at the next temperature spike. It is typically a pink, macular-papular eruption that can be faint and thus often missed. It is rarely irritating but is often more prominent in areas where the skin has been subjected to minor trauma. Generalized *lymphadenopathy* can be very florid but is particularly noticeable in the epitrochlear and axillary group. *Splenomegaly* is not such a constant feature as lymphadenopathy. Other features such as *pericarditis, pleurisy, sterile peritonitis* and *hepatitis* are less common.

The *arthritis* is a sequel to the various initial manifestations of the disease but does not occur in all cases. It usually presents as a polyarthritis of the knees, wrists, metacarpophalangeal and metatarsophalangeal joints and ankles, though not all joints will be affected at the same time. Tenosynovitis is also a feature and often the whole wrist and hand is swollen making it impossible to distinguish individual joint involvement.

The arthritis follows an unpredictable course but objective data are now emerging about prognosis in this group. It would seem that in a proportion of patients the arthritis settles without any sequelae. Others follow a chronic course of relapses and remissions. Relapses are sometimes associated with a recurrence of the systemic features and, occasionally triggered by intercurrent infections, especially of the throat.

Investigations

1. The ESR is considerably elevated, often in excess of 100mm/h.
2. A high polymorpholeucocytosis is also seen. The haemoglobin falls slowly as the disease progresses.
3. Hypergammaglobulinaemia frequently occurs but rheumatoid factors are not usually detectable in serum nor are antinuclear factors, in contradistinction to some patients with pauciarticular arthritis (*see below*).

◄ Patients are seronegative for rheumatoid factors.

4. Radiology is unhelpful diagnostically. Changes are limited to soft-tissue swelling in the initial stages. In those cases developing chronic relapsing arthritis epiphyseal growth is disturbed leading to bony deformity, and erosions are a late feature (*see* section on Radiology).

Treatment of these children is discussed in the next section on polyarticular disease.

Polyarticular disease

In this group of children emphasis is on *peripheral arthritis*. A proportion will have *systemic symptoms* initially, such as weight loss, lymphadenopathy and spiking temperatures but these features are by no means as marked as in those patients with Still's disease and a rash is very rare. There is, therefore, considerable overlap between these two groups. Girls are more commonly affected than boys and the peak age of onset is between 8 and 10. The *arthritis* is symmetrical and affects the knees, hips, wrists and small joints of the hands and feet in much the same way as in adult rheumatoid disease. In a proportion of cases early involvement of the apophyseal joints of the *cervical spine* leads to fusion and occasionally subluxation. Flexion contractures readily occur, particularly in the *hands*, and have a predilection for proximal interphalangeal joints. Involvement of the *hips* can cause considerable disability and demands rigorous and meticulous physiotherapy if later surgery is to be avoided. Linear growth impairment is almost invariable in these children. Limb growth may also become asymmetrical. Underdevelopment of the temporomandibular joint leads to a characteristic sloping chin (*micrognathism*).

◀ There is considerable clinical overlap between Still's disease and the polyarticular group.

◀ Linear growth impairment occurs invariably and limb growth may be asymmetrical.

The majority of patients are seronegative for rheumatoid factor but a small group, usually females, whose disease onset is in early teenage are seropositive and are indistinguishable from adult rheumatoid patients. The term *juvenile rheumatoid arthritis* should only be applied to this group. Development of nodules is not infrequent and the disease is often progressive demanding the early introduction of long-term disease-modifying agents such as gold and penicillamine (*see below*). Those patients who are seronegative for rheumatoid factor often remit on reaching adulthood.

◀ A small group of young female teenagers are seropositive for rheumatoid factor and indistinguishable from adult rheumatoid arthritis.

Treatment
Drugs. Salicylates in large doses are the treatment of choice. Children are surprisingly tolerant of salicylates and doses of up to 100 mg/kg body weight can be employed if necessary. Signs of toxicity (*vomiting, drowsiness* and *overbreathing*) require that the dose be reduced. Liquid aspirin preparations such as benorylate are particularly useful in young children. *Indomethacin* is also successful in controlling systemic features and joint pain and muscle spasm. Other drugs such as *naproxen* (which is also available as an elixir) can be used. *Corticosteroids* are to be avoided, chiefly because of their growth-retarding properties. They are strictly reserved for those children not responding to standard non-steroidal

◀ Children are very tolerant of salicylates.

◀ Use of steroids should be avoided as they cause serious inhibition of growth.

anti-inflammatory treatment and when systemic features of the disease, particularly the fever, continue unabated. Alternate-day dosage schedules, with the dose being given in the morning, minimize the depressant effect corticosteroids have on the hypothalamic-pituitary-adrenal axis. Symptomatic control on the day when corticosteroids are not given is achieved, although often only partially, by using increased dosages of non-steroidal anti-inflammatory medication. In some recalcitrant cases the steroid dose has to be split, i.e. high dose one day, low dose the next, to achieve acceptable symptomatic control while at the same time minimizing depressant effects on the pituitary. In other patients where systemic features are not present steroids should be avoided at all costs as side-effects, particularly growth retardation, far outweigh any therapeutic benefit. *Intra-articular corticosteroids* however, may be used cautiously in individual joints, particularly the knee.

Disease-suppressing (long-term) agents. In patients with severe persistent disease activity not controlled with standard anti-inflammatory medication, and in particular patients with seropositive juvenile rheumatoid disease, the use of disease-suppressing drugs (*see* Chapter 5) such as *gold, penicillamine* and *hydroxychloroquine* should be considered.

◄ Gold, penicillamine and hydroxychloroquine are used in those patients with severe persistent disease.

The dosage of *gold* should not exceed 1 mg/kg body weight intramuscularly weekly and test doses should be given to minimize severe allergic reactions. Treatment should continue with weekly injections until the total dose reaches approximately 1 g and then the injections spaced to fortnightly or monthly intervals. They should be continued up to at least 6 months before assessing whether there has been therapeutic benefit and provided side-effects do not supervene (*see* Chapter 5). If there has been a therapeutic response maintenance treatment with monthly or 2-monthly injections should be instituted and continued indefinitely, side-effects permitting.

Penicillamine has also been used in children but experience is still limited and dosage regimes not fully worked out. *Hydrochloroquine* in a dosage of 7 mg/kg body weight daily can also be used as a disease-suppressing therapy although in general it is less successful than either gold or penicillamine. Complications are the same as for adult usage and regular eye checks are mandatory. Maintenance dose should be kept as low as possible and usually an alternate-day regime is sufficient in younger children. Courses of the drug should not exceed 2 years.

Immunosuppressive therapy with either azathioprine, cyclophosphamide or chlorambucil should only be resorted to in extreme cases because of the possible mutagenic and oncogenic effects which are more likely in children. However, in patients with severe systemic and/or seropositive disease who develop amyloidosis immunosuppressive therapy may be life-saving (*see below*).

Physiotherapy. This is a vital part of any treatment regime used in childhood arthritis. Contractures and muscle wasting occur with alarming rapidity in children if scrupulous care is not taken to avoid them. *Hydrotherapy* is particularly valuable. Splinting of joints is sometimes necessary to prevent deformities and is used in conjunction with active and passive physiotherapy. *Resting splints* for night use are especially indicated in the treatment of knee and hip contractures to promote correct posture when at rest. Prone lying for periods during the day in children with hip involvement helps prevent contractures which can be particularly insidious at the hip joint.

Rest. Complete bed rest is occasionally indicated in patients with acute arthritis and systemic involvement but should be kept to a minimum and passive physiotherapy applied to joints to prevent contractures. There is little doubt that acute arthritis will settle during a period of rest but it is imperative that this is not at the expense of irreversible joint contractures that may ensue. A modified rest regime including short periods out of bed usually with the physiotherapist, and allowing the child up to the toilet is often the best course of action. In less acute cases the child can be allowed to be as active as he or she likes and it is in any case often impossible and sometimes counter-productive to inflict strict regimes.

◄ Even during periods of bed rest passive physiotherapy is used to prevent joint contractures.

Social aspects. These are extremely important and it is essential that a good rapport is built up between not only the children but also their parents who have to shoulder a good deal of responsibility in the management of chronic arthritis. Time is a precious commodity in the life of children and as much attention should be applied to their mental and psychological well-being as to their physical well-being. Schooling can continue during inevitable periods of hospitalization which should be kept to a minimum. It may be necessary to send the child to a special school where expert physiotherapy, including hydrotherapy, is available, but even in these cases every effort should be made to ensure as normal life a for the child as the disease allows.

Surgery. Soft-tissue release operations and osteotomy may be required to correct severe deformities but in general surgery should be postponed as long as possible at least until early teenage or when growth has ceased. Hip arthroplasty is now well established in the treatment of juveniles with hip deformities, particularly in females with adduction deformities which have proved unresponsive to conservative corrective techniques. Advances in surgical technique, particularly in the field of joint replacement, will pay handsome dividends in this fortunately small group of patients.

Pauciarticular disease
As the title suggests, this term is applied to those children with a small number of joints involved (*four or less*), often presenting as a monoarthritis. This is probably the most difficult group to define as some cases of polyarticular disease can present with a pauciarticular arthritis and subsequently develop other joint involvement and thus have to be re-defined.

The arthritis tends to affect the lower limb joints but any joint including the cervical spine can be involved. It often results in severe growth abnormalities of the affected limbs.

These children are seronegative for rheumatoid factor but some have positive *antinuclear factors* in their serum (with negative DNA binding). This group are particularly prone to develop chronic iridocyclitis (anterior uveitis). This can be sight threatening and has several manifestations. Onset is usually insidious and therefore regular ophthalmological monitoring, including slit lamp examination of the anterior chamber, is mandatory. The initial changes are of pus in the anterior chamber and

◄ Children with pauci-articular disease and positive ANF are at risk from chronic iridocyclitis.

precipitates on the back of the cornea — *keratic precipitates*. The cornea can undergo secondary degeneration as the eye lesions progress and produces a characteristic *band keratopathy* which is often visible with the naked eye. Posterior and anterior *synechiae* form and may result in an irregular pupil and secondary *glaucoma*. *Cataracts* also form. Treatment with mydriatics and topical steroids is vital if sight is to be preserved. In some cases of persistent iridocyclitis treatment with immunosuppressive therapy is under investigation. Constant vigilance is essential in monitoring the eyes of these patients with pauciarticular disease, and those with a positive ANF should have slit lamp examination every 3 months. Occasionally patients with systemic polyarthritic disease also develop iridocyclitis, another example of overlap between the various groups.

◀ Three-monthly ocular monitoring is mandatory in ANF-positive pauciarticular disease.

Juvenile ankylosing spondylitis
A predominantly male sub-group with pauci-articular disease, the majority of whom are HLA B27 positive (*see* Chapter 7), eventually develop *ankylosing spondylitis*. The joints initially involved are the knees, hips and ankles, often asymmetric-ally. The age of onset varies but it is unusual before the age of 9 and reaches a maximum in the early teens. The disease has all the characteristics of adult ankylosing spondylitis including enthesopathies, uveitis and, rarely, aortitis.

◀ The subgroup of B27 positive males with pauciarticular disease may develop ankylosing spondylitis.

Serious spinal involvement does not occur until adulthood. This often means that the diagnosis in childhood has to be presumptive rather than definite. A *family history* of the disease is of vital diagnostic importance. Treatment is the same as for the adult disease.

Amyloidosis in juvenile chronic arthritis
This is a serious complication of juvenile chronic arthritis affecting some 7–8% of patients. It is more common in those children with *relapsing systemic disease* and *polyarthritis*. It is heralded by asymp-tomatic *proteinuria* and the diagnosis is made by either *rectal* or, if necessary, *renal biopsy*. Treatment is unsatisfactory and the best hope of survival is to

◀ Amyloidosis is more common in children with relapsing systemic disease and polyarthritis.

control the systemic disease or for it to go into spontaneous remission. *Chlorambucil* seems to benefit some patients with amyloidosis but in general the outlook is poor. Most deaths are caused by renal failure and/or intercurrent infection.

The radiology of juvenile chronic arthritis

This has already been mentioned in the section on systemic juvenile arthritis. *Growth abnormalities* are the most common radiological signs of the disease as epiphyseal maturation is affected by the adjacent arthritis. This is particularly so in pauciarticular disease, especially around the knee joint but can be seen around any affected joint. *Juxta-articular osteoporosis* and osteoporosis of long bones due to disuse atrophy are also commonly seen. *Bony erosions* are a late manifestation of the disease as the articular cartilage in children is thicker than it is in adults. *Fusion* of the apophyseal joints of the *cervical spine*, sometimes with atlanto-axial subluxation, is a characteristic radiological feature in some children with polyarticular disease. In juvenile ankylosing spondylitis radiological change of the sacro-iliac joint is a late feature and interpretation of these joints is notoriously difficult in children.

◀ Bony erosions are a late manifestation of juvenile chronic arthritis.

Further Reading

Ansell, Barbara M. (1980) *Rheumatic Disorders in Childhood*. Postgraduate Paediatrics Series. London, Butterworths.

Some other conditions causing arthropathy and musculoskeletal pain **13**

Many general medical conditions may present, or be associated with, musculoskeletal pain including arthritis and arthralgia. Some of the more important ones are discussed briefly in this chapter. They serve to illustrate the diversity of disease that may present at a rheumatology clinic.

Endocrine disorders

Acromegaly

Joint pain and swelling in acromegaly are not uncommon. It has several causes:
- Chondrocalcinosis and pseudogout
- Premature osteoarthritis
- Juxta-articular periostitis
- Degenerative disease of the spine resulting in ankylosing hyperostosis

One of the characteristic radiological features of acromegaly, apart from bony hypertrophy, is an apparent widening of the joint spaces, particularly in the fingers. There is also an increased incidence of carpal tunnel and other entrapment neuropathies.

◄ Acromegaly causes widening of the radiological joint spaces.

Thyrotoxicosis and hypothyroidism

- Thyrotoxicosis may be associated with a proximal myopathy
- Digital clubbing and periostitis can occur in thyrotoxicosis — this is known as *thyroid acropachy*

◄ Thyroid acropachy (finger clubbing and periostitis) occurs in thyrotoxicosis.

- Chondrocalcinosis and pseudogout occur in hypothyroidism
- There is an increased incidence of thyroid disease in rheumatoid arthritis

Cushing's syndrome (including iatrogenic Cushing's)
- Osteoporotic vertebral collapse and fractures in the distal skeleton
- A rare mutilating arthropathy occurring in untreated Cushing's syndrome as a consequence of ligamentous laxity and aseptic necrosis of bone

Diabetes
- Chondrocalcinosis is said to be more common in diabetes
- Diabetic neuropathy can result in severe painless destructive osteoarthritis (Charcot's joints) — originally described in syphilitic neuropathy (tabes dorsalis)

◄ Diabetic peripheral neuropathy may lead to severe painless osteoarthritis, i.e. Charcot's joints.

Hyperparathyroidism
- Chondrocalcinosis and pseudogout
- Metabolic bone disease — osteoporosis and fractures
- As a cause of renal failure resulting in hyperuricaemia and secondary gout
- Rarely, a peripheral erosive synovitis.

Blood disorders

Haemophilic arthropathy
Patients with haemophilia may bleed into their joints (haemarthrosis) and more frequently into the surrounding soft tissues. In the case of haemarthrosis this may be associated with trauma or occur spontaneously. Recurrent haemarthroses lead to destruction of articular cartilage and fibrous contractures within the joints and a mutilating chronic

◄ Recurrent haemarthroses in haemophilia can cause severe destructive joint changes.

arthritis. The knees are most commonly affected but any synovial joint may become involved. Prompt treatment is essential if chronic haemophilic arthropathy is not to result. The basis of treatment is as follows:

◄ Haemophilic arthritis can be very destructive — prompt treatment is vital.

1. Oral or parenteral analgesia (haemarthrosis is extremely painful)
2. Infusion of cryoprecipitate to correct the deficient clotting factors
3. Aspiration of the joint if a painful, tense effusion occurs
4. Physiotherapy to maintain muscle strength and prevent joint contractures

Haemoglobinopathies

Sickle-cell disease is the chief cause of arthropathy in this group. It affects the joints and bones in several ways:

1. In an acute sickle-cell crisis, arthralgia and/or synovitis is common
2. Infarction of bone occurs due to thrombosis of the nutrient vessels. This results in aseptic necrosis of bone

◄ Sickle-cell disease may result in bone infarction, aseptic necrosis and osteomyelitis.

3. Septic arthritis and/or osteomyelitis — the usual infecting organism is salmonella (*see* Chapter 11)
4. Periostitis resulting in painful tender digits, i.e. dactylitis

Leukaemia

All the leukaemias may be complicated by an arthropathy and/or bone pain and musculoskeletal symptoms are common in this group of diseases. There are several causes:

1. Leukaemic infiltration of the synovium leads to synovitis and effusion. Leukaemic cells can be identified in the synovial fluid aspirated from such joints
2. Secondary hyperuricaemia and gout
3. Bony deposits causing bone pain and pathological fractures
4. Haemarthroses due to a bleeding disorder, usually thrombocytopenia

Multiple myeloma
Musculoskeletal manifestations of this disease are:
1. Bone pain, pathological fractures (particularly of the lumbar vertebra) due to plasma cell infiltration
2. Osteoporosis
3. Amyloid deposition in the synovium which may cause an arthropathy resembling a rheumatoid arthritis
4. Carpal tunnel syndrome due to amyloid deposition beneath the flexor retinaculum
5. Secondary gout as the result of hyperuricaemia
6. Multiple myeloma is more common in patients with rheumatoid arthritis

◀ Amyloid arthropathy occurring in multiple myeloma mimics rheumatoid arthritis.

Cryoglobulinaemia
This may complicate several blood dyscrasias, particularly lymphomas. The cryoglobulins produced in these conditions cause Raynaud's phenomenon (*see* Chapter 6).

Hypogammaglobulinaemia
Deficiency (hypogammaglobulinaemia) or complete lack of gammaglobulins (agammaglobulinaemia) can be either congenital or acquired. Several congenital types have now been described. Whatever the cause, the patients are susceptible to bacterial infections and septic arthritis. They may also suffer a non-specific synovitis which may be associated with diarrhoea and malabsorption. Occasionally the synovitis may be symmetrical and indistinguishable from rheumatoid arthritis and cartilage erosion may occur. Tests for rheumatoid factor are negative.

Musculoskeletal disorders associated with malignancy

Hypertrophic pulmonary osteoarthropathy (HPOA)
In this condition there is synovitis and periostitis usually seen at the wrists and the ankles, though the

synovitis may affect any synovial joint. It may present as an oligoarthritis. Patients not only complain of painful joints but also of tender bones, particularly around the wrist and ankle joints. Tenderness may be elicited on palpation around the lower radius and tibia. This is due to *periostitis*. *Clubbing* may also be associated. Radiographs show typical subperiosteal new bone formation. The commonest cause is bronchial carcinoma, but other causes are listed below — note not all involve the lung:

◀ The commonest cause of HPOA is carcinoma of the lung.

1. Chronic suppurative lung disease, e.g. bronchiectasis, empyema
2. Cyanotic heart disease
3. Pulmonary metastatic disease
4. Pulmonary tuberculosis
5. Crohn's disease and ulcerative colitis
6. Cirrhosis
7. Intestinal lymphoma

Carcinomatous myopathy
This can be associated with any malignancy, but especially with bronchial carcinoma and squamous-cell carcinomas, e.g. oesophagus. Proximal muscle weakness, general malaise and weight loss are the cardinal signs. Muscle enzymes are usually normal and electromyographic studies non-specific. Successful treatment of the primary lesion may result in resolution of the myopathy but in general these patients carry a poor prognosis.

◀ Carcinomatous myopathy carries a poor prognosis.

Dermatomyositis and polymyositis
Approximately 10% of patients over the age of 40 with these conditions are found to have an underlying malignancy. The most common association is with carcinoma of the lung, ovary, prostate and gut (*see* Chapter 6).

Malignant synovitis
A non-specific synovitis can complicate malignant disease (usually disseminated). In some respects this could be regarded as a reactive arthritis as direct invasion of the synovium is not seen in the majority of cases. Occasionally the juxta-articular bone may show secondary deposits.

Bone pain. Bony metastases are very frequent in a variety of tumours, particularly bronchus, breast, kidney, thyroid, bowel and prostate. Patients may present with local bone pain particularly in the spine (*see* Chapter 3). Pathological fractures may occur.

Tumours of the synovium
These are rare and strict pathological classification is complicated. There are basically two types:

1. Malignant synovioma. This is a rare, highly malignant tumour originating from synovial cells, derived from either the joints or tendon sheaths. It presents as a monoarticular swelling and can occur in or around any synovial joint or tendon sheath, but it is most commonly found in the extremities, particularly around the knees and ankles but the small joints of the hands may be involved. The juxta-articular swelling may be present for several years before pain alerts the patient to seek medical advice. Occasionally patients present with breathlessness and haemoptysis signifying pulmonary metastases. Haemarthroses also occur. Prognosis is poor.

2. Pigmented villonodular synovitis. This is a benign lesion and presents as a swelling of synovial joints, particularly the knees. Occasionally severe pain may occur usually signifying a haemarthrosis. The tumour comprises a mass of hypertrophied synovial tissue that forms fronds (villi) within the joint. It has a brown colour due to repeated haemorrhage and deposits of haemosiderin in synovial cells and surrounding tissues. Local invasion of cartilage and bone is invariable. Secondary osteoarthritis may supervene. Treatment is by excision and/or radio-synovectomy. Recurrence rate is high. Diagnosis rests on synovial biopsy and this can be readily achieved by arthroscopy.

Sarcoidosis
This is a granulomatous disease of unknown aetiology which is more common in Negroes than in Caucasians. It is more prevalent in Scandinavia than in other European countries. An arthritis is not an uncommon complication and occurs in approximately 30% of patients. It is of two types, both being more common in women than in men.

◄ Sarcoid arthritis occurs in 30% of patients, and may be either acute and non-destructive or chronic and destructive.

1. Acute symmetrical migratory polyarthritis. This is self-limiting and associated with other systemic features of sarcoidosis which it may antedate:
- Erythema nodosum
- Hilar lymphadenopathy and pulmonary infiltrates (90%)
- Uveitis
- Fever
- Tenosynovitis and tendonitis
- Rarely, sacro-iliitis
- Myopathy (rarely)

2. A chronic arthritis that may be destructive. This type is associated with sarcoid granulomas within the synovium, the juxta-articular bone and elsewhere in the body. It is much rarer than the acute arthritis but far more significant in terms of deleterious effect on joint function.

Further Reading
Huskisson E. C. and Hart F. Dudley (1978) *Joint Disease: all the Arthropathies*. Bristol, Wright

History and examination of the musculoskeletal system

14

In this chapter the basic techniques of history taking and examination applied to patients with musculoskeletal complaints are explained. It is impossible to cover every nuance of technique in such a chapter because this has to be learned in the consulting room and at the bedside.

The history

The art of good history taking is to obtain diagnostically relevant information as quickly and as accurately as possible. The mechanical listing of answers to questions without due thought as to their diagnostic significance is a tendency which should be avoided at all costs. *You must have a reason for asking a question.* It is always useful to have a framework of questions worked out for all patients and modify it accordingly as your diagnostic 'nose' develops. The following question list may be useful in this respect. It may seem daunting at first reading but, with practice, students should be able to pick out the relevant information as they go along and be prepared to switch their line of questioning.

The introduction

This should always include the patient's age, sex and occupation. This not only provides important diagnostic information but with these simple questions it is often possible to allay some of the patient's anxiety and fears.

The presenting complaint

Pain is the most common presenting symptom in musculoskeletal diseases and much diagnostic information can be gleaned from a patient's description of the pain. The relevant information that is required, much of which will be spontaneously given by the patient, is encapsulated in the following list of questions.

1. Where? — Try to pin the patient down to the exact site of maximum intensity of the pain. In peripheral arthritis it is usually centred over a joint. In back pain and soft-tissue rheumatism the patient is often unable to be specific but is usually able to indicate the general area of pain. *Radiating* pain is always important diagnostically. The more common conditions, which can give rise to radiating pain are shown in *Table* 14.1.

2. How long? — It is important to get as accurate assessment of the duration of pain as possible. Prompting questions such as 'Is it days, weeks, months or years?' usually help in those patients who seem to have lost all sense of time.

3. Onset — acute or chronic? — The acute onset of *traumatic* musculoskeletal pain is usually remembered vividly. *Inflammatory* pain usually builds up to a crescendo over a few days, although occasionally patients with acute *rheumatoid arthritis* describe the joint pain as coming on very suddenly. The excruciating pain of *gout* often comes on during the night, waking the patient from his sleep. The pain of *osteoarthritis* usually builds up over a number of years and is sometimes described as 'my rheumatics'.

Table 14.1.   Causes of radiating pain

1. Hip synovitis (to ipsilateral knee)
2. Sacro-iliitis (to groin, buttock and posterior thigh)
3. Sciatica (in dermatome distribution)
4. Costovertebral (around rib cage and anterior chest)
5. Cervical spondylosis (shoulder girdle, in dermatomes of arm)
6. Shoulder capsulitis (to outer aspect of upper arm)
7. Bicipital tendinitis (into muscle belly of biceps)
8. Tennis elbow (into forearm)
9. Carpal tunnel syndrome (median nerve distribution and up to elbow)

4. Timing of pain? — This is particularly relevant in inflammatory pain which is often worse early morning on waking and is sometimes present after a period of inactivity such as sitting for any length of time. The former is known as *early morning stiffness* and the latter as *inactivity stiffness*. This stiffness can often be 'worked off'. The joint stiffness of rheumatoid arthritis exhibits just these characteristics. The early morning limb girdle muscular stiffness occurring in elderly patients, often female, is one of the cardinal features of *polymyalgia rheumatica*. Similarly the early morning back stiffness experienced by young males with *ankylosing spondylitis* can be a vital diagnostic clue.

◄ Inflammatory pain is often worse in the early morning. Joints may be 'stiff' — early morning stiffness.

5. Any relieving or exacerbating factors? — E.g. warmth, cold, activity, inactivity. Do particular movements make the pain worse?

6. Have there been any previous episodes of similar pain? — Previous history of pain is especially important in rheumatic diseases as many of them relapse and remit. This is especially relevant in rheumatoid arthritis and ankylosing spondylitis as previous episodes, possibly not as acute as the presenting one, may have been ignored by the patient, but help to date the onset of disease which may have important therapeutic implications.

7. How would you describe your pain? — Many patients embark on long detailed descriptions of their pain during which diagnostic clues can sometimes be gleaned. A few of the many that should alert your attention are:
  a. 'Like a door creaking' — old lady with severe osteoarthritis of the knees.
  b. 'Just like walking on pebbles' — young woman with rheumatoid arthritis and severe arthritis of the metatarsophalangeal joints.
  c. 'It is as though my back is in a vice' — man with ankylosing spondylitis.
  d. 'Like cotton wool', 'tingling', 'numbness', 'coldness', 'burning' — tend to suggest neurological involvement, e.g. rheumatoid neuropathy.
  e. 'Excruciating, I can't even bear the weight of the bed clothes on my foot' — patient with gout.

Assessment of function

Apart from pain it is the loss of joint function that most affects patients and an enquiry into overall *functional capacity* of each patient must be made. This should be very simple but relevant. A few examples of useful questions are listed here:
1. Can you dress yourself unaided?
2. Can you bath yourself unaided?
3. Do you have any difficulty in the kitchen? e.g. lifting pots and pans, peeling potatoes, etc.
4. Do you have difficulty at work? e.g. using tools, lifting objects, etc.
5. Can you climb up and down stairs unaided?
6. Are any everyday tasks difficult to perform? e.g. opening doors, writing, getting in and out of a chair, etc.

Some associated symptoms relevant to rheumatological conditions

1. Is there any history of rashes? If so, what sort. Psoriasis and the photosensitive butterfly rash of SLE are particularly relevant in this regard.
2. Any symptoms of *cold sensitivity*, i.e. Raynaud's phenomenon (particularly experienced by patients with SLE and scleroderma but also seen in rheumatoid arthritis).
3. Has there been any inflammation of the eyes or any pain in the eyes? (*scleritis* — rheumatoid arthritis; *uveitis* — ankylosing spondylitis; *conjunctivitis* — Reiter's syndrome).
4. Do you experience any grittiness of the eyes or dryness of the mouth? (*Sjögren's syndrome*).
5. Has there been any loss of hair? (*alopecia* in SLE).
6. Have you experienced any change in *bowel habit*? Have you had an attack of diarrhoea recently? (enteropathic arthritis, Reiter's syndrome).

General systemic enquiry

Symptomatic enquiries into all the systems must be undertaken so that an impression of the patient's general health may be gained.

Family history
A positive family history is not uncommon in *rheumatoid arthritis.* 'Is there any arthritis in your family?' 'Do any of your relatives suffer from joint deformities?' *Ankylosing spondylitis* has a strong familial association. 'Is there any back trouble in your family?' 'Does anyone walk with a stoop, or have a stiff neck?' Other diseases such as *psoriasis* and *colitis* present in the family are highly relevant. In patients with *osteoarthritis* a family history is almost inevitable as it is such a common disease. Certain types of osteoarthritis, particularly *primary Heberden's node-positive osteoarthritis* in females, follow an inherited pattern. *Gout* patients too often exhibit a positive family history.

Drug history
It is important to establish which particular drug(s) the patient has been taking, including proprietary preparations. Most will have tried at least one anti-inflammatory preparation and many will have taken a variety. Any side-effects, such as *indigestion* or *skin rash*, must be carefully documented.

The Examination
All patients should first have a *general examination* before examination of the musculoskeletal system is undertaken as many so-called 'rheumatic conditions' are secondary to generalized disease (*see* Chapter 13).
Many joint diseases give rise to physical signs outside the musculoskeletal system, e.g. *spleno-megaly, lymphadenopathy, scleritis, vasculitic ulcers, peripheral neuropathy*, all occurring in *rheumatoid arthritis; aortic incompetence*, occurring in *ankylosing spondylitis; systemic lupus erythematosus* and its protean clinical manifestations. These are just a few examples that serve to make the point that unless a general examination is performed, many important clinical signs will be missed.

◄ A general examination should always be performed in addition to a musculoskeletal examination.

Examination of the musculoskeletal system
Examination of the musculoskeletal system must follow the same logical sequence as examination of

any other system with a few particular exceptions. Although most of the examination will be devoted to the joints, it must not be forgotten that joints are activated by muscles and these should also be carefully examined. The following scheme should be adopted:

1. Inspection
2. Palpation
3. Assessment of active movement
4. Assessment of passive movement
5. Assessment of function

A full musculoskeletal survey, once the techniques have been mastered, should take no more than *5 min*.

1. Inspection

The following features should be noted:

a. Is the joint correctly *aligned*? i.e. does it lie normally in its position of rest (*neutral position*). If it deviates from this position then this should be noted.

   i. Deviation from the vertical axis at the *knee, elbow* and *ankle* is known as *valgus* (away from the midline) or *varus* (towards the midline).

   ii. At the hip vertical deviation is described as *abduction* (away from the midline) or *adduction* (towards the midline).

   iii. In the hands and wrists, vertical deviation is described as either *ulnar* or *radial*.

   iv. Deviation in the *horizontal axis* is described in terms of *flexion* or *extension* with the exception of the *ankles* and *toes* which can be either *dorsiflexed* or *plantarflexed*

The extent of the deformity should be estimated in terms of degree of deviation from the neutral position. Exact measurement is not usually necessary unless response to a particular physiotherapy regime, such as correction of fixed flexion deformity of the knee, is to be assessed or the deformity is to be corrected surgically.

b. Is the joint swollen?
c. Is the joint red? } indicating inflammation.
d. Is the joint warm?

2. Palpation

The key note in this part of the examination is to be gentle but firm. The basic signs one is seeking are as follows:

a. Is the joint warm? It is usually customary to use the back of the examining hand to assess this as the palm tends to be warmer.

b. If the joint is swollen, is the swelling soft tissue, bone or fluid? Does it fluctuate?

c. Is the joint tender? A firm squeeze is all that is required and this should be done whilst *looking at the patient* to assess his response. This can be a *wince*, a *cry* or a *rapid withdrawal* of the inflamed area from the examining hand, depending on the severity of the inflammation. If, on inspection, the signs of acute inflammation, i.e. redness and swelling, are obvious then eliciting tenderness should be performed with extreme caution.

d. Is there crepitus within the joint? This can be palpable and/or audible. It usually denotes damage to the articular sufaces of the joint and in these cases has a coarse quality. It may also emanate from the soft tissues, particularly the synovium in rheumatoid arthritis when it is a much finer and superficial quality.

e. Extra-articular signs help such as palpable although invisible nodules over bony prominences in rheumatoid arthritis.

Muscle tenderness and thickened skin should also be noted during the course of palpation.

3. Assessment of active movement

What degree of voluntary movement are the joints capable of? Thus the patient is asked to put each joint through its full range of movement and any diminution of this range is noted and roughly estimated. In the case of the hand this can be simplified by asking the patient to:

a. Make a fist

b. Stretch his fingers apart

c. Pinch his thumb and little finger together

4. Assessment of passive movement

Often the *active range* of movement around a joint is less than the *passive range*, i.e. the range achieved when the joint is moved gently but firmly by the examiner. This is particularly so in the fingers when active movement may be limited by damaged tendons or dislocated (subluxed) joints. As in active movement the degree of any restriction in a particular direction should be estimated.

◄ Assessment of movement requires that the patient be relaxed; this requires a confident yet sympathetic approach from the examiner.

5. *Assessment of function*

This is most important, though it is impossible to perform a full functional assessment of the musculo-skeletal system during a standard examination. During the history taking limitation of function around certain joints should have been highlighted. These can be assessed first hand in the examination room by observing the patient during manoeuvres such as:

a. Walking across the examination room. Is the patient walking unaided or is he using a stick or a walking frame? Does he have modified foot wear?

b. Undressing and dressing.

c. Getting on and off the couch.

d. Getting into and out of a chair.

Examination of individual joints

The approach to examination of individual joints should be planned in a logical fashion otherwise important physical signs will be missed. Whatever plan you adopt it should be simple and straight-forward and well practised. The following scheme is only a suggestion as to how the examination should proceed.

1. Examination of the hands and wrists
2. Examination of the elbows
3. Examination of the shoulders
4. Examination of the neck
5. Examination of the hips
6. Examination of the knees
7. Examination of the ankles
8. Examination of the subtalar joints
9. Examination of the metatarsophalangeal joints
10. Examination of the thoracic and lumbar spine and the sacro-iliac joints

Examination of the hands and wrists

Inspection of the hands is best performed with them resting comfortably on a desk top or in the patient's lap. Both the palmar and extensor aspects should be examined. The following diagram illustrates some of the important signs to be found in the hands — further details are found in the preceding text and *Fig.* 14.1 should serve as a revision exercise.

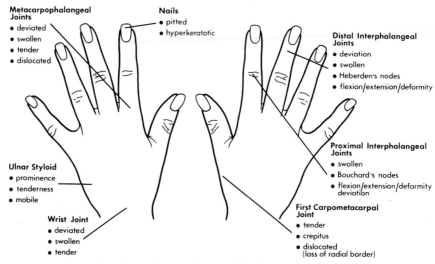

Fig. 14.1. Joint signs in the hand in rheumatic disease.

Examination of the elbows

Movements possible at the elbow are:
a. Flexion
b. Extension } at the humero-ulnar joint.
c. Pronation and supination (at the superior radio-ulnar joint).

Special points to note are:
a. Presence or absence of a fixed flexion deformity.
b. Crepitus, particularly on pronation and supination (best felt with the examining fingers over the radial head whilst the forearm is passively pronated and supinated).
c. Presence or absence of rheumatoid nodules, either over the olecranon and/or extending down the ulna.
d. An olecranon bursa may be present.
e. The elbow is a site of predilection for psoriatic plaques and these may be very small.

Examination of the shoulders

This is best done with the patient seated on a low-back chair. Do not forget that the shoulder comprises three components:
a. Clavicle
b. Scapula } acromioclavicular joint.
c. Glenohumeral joint.

The movements possible at this joint are:
a. Abduction
b. Adduction

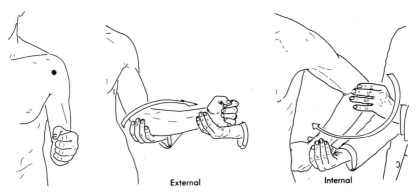

External   Internal

Fig. 14.2.   External and internal rotation of shoulder.

c. Flexion
d. Extension
e. Internal rotation ⎫
f. External rotation ⎭ *see Fig.* 14.2

The first four of these movements are achieved not only by movement at the scapular humeral joint but also by displacement of the scapula itself (*Fig.* 14.3). *Passive abduction* is best tested by standing behind the patient and fixing the infralateral border of the scapula within the thumb and abducting the arm. Any movement of the scapula before 90° abduction is indicative of an adhesive capsulitis (*frozen shoulder*). This is discussed in more detail in Chapter 1 as is the concept of '*the painful arc*'.

◀ Any movement of the scapula before 90° of abduction of the shoulder is indicative of a 'frozen shoulder'.

During palpation of the shoulder joint the following areas should receive particular attention:
a. Tenderness at or just below the corocoid process indicating inflammation with the glenohumeral joint itself.
b. Tenderness over the humeral bicipital groove indicating tendinitis of the long head of biceps.
c. Tenderness over the acromioclavicular joints indicating a synovitis within them, e.g. rheumatoid arthritis, ankylosing spondylitis.
d. Tenderness just below the lateral border of the acromion indicating a supraspinatus tendinitis or bursitis.

In addition to noting swelling, redness and any changes in contour, muscle bulk should also be assessed, i.e. is there any wasting? any winging of the scapula (denoting profound muscle weakness or neurological damage)?

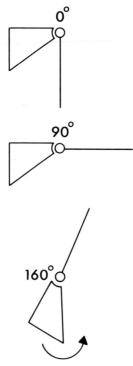

Fig. 14.3. Diagrammatic representation of shoulder abduction. Note scapula rotation.

Examination of the cervical spine

Again this is best achieved with the patient sitting. The attitude of the head should be noted. Movements to be tested are (*Fig.* 14.4):

a. Forward flexion ('put your chin on your chest')
b. Extension ('look to the ceiling')
c. Lateral flexion ('touch your right/left shoulder with your right/left ear')
d. Rotation
e. Crepitus may be elicited by palpation over the spinous processes and may even be audible. It usually indicates damage to the posterior apophyseal joints or to the atlanto-axial articulation which is commonly involved in rheumatoid arthritis

Both active and passive movements should be assessed, and examination of the neck should always include a neurological examination of the arms (*see* Chapter 4).

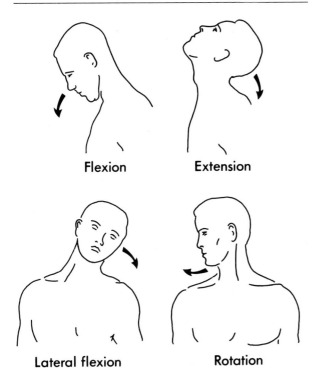

Flexion   Extension

Lateral flexion   Rotation

Fig. 14.4.   Movements of the cervical spine.

Examination of the hips

This should be performed with the patient lying flat and the attitude of the legs should be noted. Are they held:

a. Flexed (mild flexion deformity can be compensated for by the patient increasing his lumbar lordosis (*Fig.* 14.5)

b. Abducted

c. Adducted

d. Internally or externally rotated (look at the position of the foot)

Movements of the hips are (*Fig.*14.6):

a. Flexion

b. Extension

c. Abduction

e. Adduction

f. Internal rotation

g. External rotation

When testing *flexion* it is important to observe the behaviour of the opposite hip. Failure to do this will result in missing a mild *flexion deformity*. A hand

◀ A fixed flexion deformity at the hip can be masked by the patient increasing his lumbar lordosis and be missed by the examiner unless Thomas' test is applied.

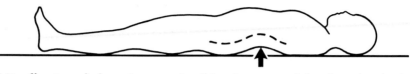

Hip flexion deformity masked by increased lumbar lordosis

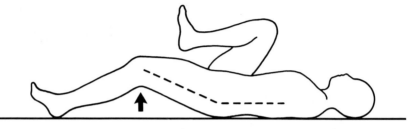

Hip flexion deformity unmasked by flexion of opposite hip

Fig. 14.5. Thomas' test for fixed flexion deformity of the hip. Note patient adopts exaggerated lumbar lordosis to allow affected limb to rest on couch. For full explanation *see* text.

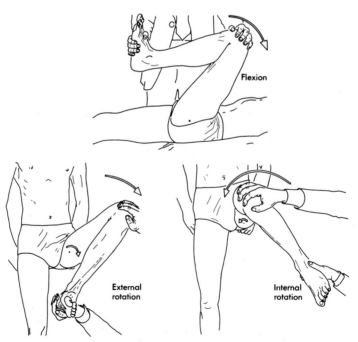

Fig. 14.6. Testing flexion, internal and external rotation at the hip.

should be placed under the lumbar spine and the hip flexed as fully as possible. If a flexion deformity is present in the opposite hip, that hip will be seen to rise from the couch as the patient flattens his exaggerated lumbar lordosis and allows his pelvis to rotate upwards, thus lifting the fixed hip off the couch, this is known as Thomas' test (*see Fig.* 14.5). Fixed flexion deformity of one hip will produce *apparent shortening* of the leg as will adduction or abduction deformities.

◄ Deformities at the hip joint may lead to apparent shortening of the leg.

Examination of the knees
Movements of the knee joint are:
a. Flexion
b. Extension
c. Internal rotation ⎫
d. External rotation ⎭ with the joint flexed
Deformities of the joint are:
a. Flexion deformity
b. Abduction (genu valgum)
c. Adduction (genu varus)
Occasionally the knee may be held in *hyperextension*.

Inspection. With the patient supine the knee should be examined for:
1. Muscle wasting, particularly of the quadriceps
2. Deformities (as above)
3. Effusion (disappearance of the suprapatellar dimples)
   Particular attention should be paid to any swellings in the popliteal fossa (Baker's cyst).

Detection of a knee-joint effusion. Effusion of the knee joint is detected by the standard method of *fluctuation*. Fluid tends to accumulate in the suprapatellar pouch and this is first pushed into the knee joint itself by gentle downwards pressure; the joint is then fluctuated by the other hand by squeezing on the medial and lateral aspects of the joint. Smaller amounts of fluid may be detected by pressure over the lateral aspect of the joint, pushing fluid over to the medial compartment and then with a gentle stroking action the fluid is pushed back to the lateral side of the joint, distending the lateral suprapatellar dimple. If sufficient fluid is present a *patellar tap* may be elicited. During this test fluid is squeezed out of the suprapatellar pouch with one hand

and with the other hand the patella is 'tapped' down on to the patella–femoral articulation. For this test to be positive considerable fluid has to be present.

It should be remembered that effusion is not always due to synovial fluid but other fluids such as *blood* and *pus* will give identical physical signs, and positive identification can only be made by needle aspiration of the joint (arthrocentesis).

Testing for stability. As in all other diarthrodial joints, the stability of the knee joint is dependent on:
1. Integrity of the articular cartilage and subchondral bone.
2. The muscles acting around the joint; in the case of the knee joint the quadriceps muscles are most important in this respect.
3. The ligaments (these are particularly important at the knee joint and at the ankle joint).

Anteroposterior stability. The very powerful cruciate ligaments are chiefly responsible for maintaining anteroposterior stability of the knee joint. Damage to them, resulting in either rupture or laxity, allows the tibia to be pulled forwards and pushed backwards on the femoral articulation with the knee flexed and the foot placed firmly on the couch (*Fig.* 14.7).

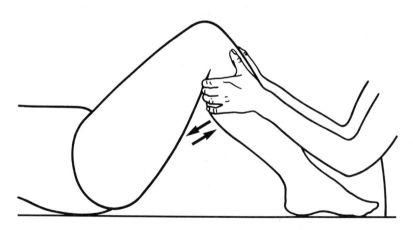

Testing the cruciate ligaments

Fig. 14.7. Testing for laxity of the cruciate ligaments.

Testing for medial and lateral stability. To test for the integrity of the medial and lateral collateral ligaments of the knee joint the leg is fully extended and held at the ankle beneath the examiner's arm. The lower leg is then forcibly abducted and adducted. At full extension the knee joint should be locked and no movement possible and movement in either a medial or lateral direction, or both, signifies not only laxity of the collateral ligaments but also loss of cartilage and/or bone in either the medial or lateral compartments of the knee.

◀ Loss of cartilage and bone is often a major contributory factor to knee joint instability, particularly in the more destructive forms of arthritis.

Testing movements. Testing flexion and extension at the knee joint is straight forward. Care must be taken to lay a hand over the patella while passive flexion and extension movements are performed as knee joint crepitus can be readily elicited in this way. The *patella* is usually mobile and can be displaced medially, laterally and to a certain extent, superiorly and inferiorly with the quadriceps muscle suitably relaxed. Whilst testing these movements firm downward pressure on the patella may elicit a *retropatellar tenderness* either due to synovitis or to damage of the patellar cartilage. Such damage occurs in osteoarthritis and a condition chiefly found in young women called *chondromalacia patellae* which results in roughening of the retropatellar cartilage.

◀ Retropatellar tenderness in a young woman may signify chondromalacia patellae.

Rotation is strictly limited at the knee joint but what few degrees there are are very important for knee joint function. 'Unlocking' of the knee joint from the fully extended position requires rotation of the tibial plateaux on the femoral condyles. Rotation of the joint is limited by the attachments of the medial and lateral menisci, by the ligaments and muscles. To test rotation of the knee joint, the joint is slightly flexed and the ankle is firmly grasped and the tibia rotated either externally or internally.

To test for the integrity of the menisci the joint is flexed and fixed alternately in external and internal rotation (by twisting at the ankle) and then *slowly* extended. Pain during this movement, or an audible or palpable clunk or click is indicative of a torn meniscus. This is known as *McMurray's test*.

◀ McMurray's test is used to assess the integrity of the knee menisci.

Examination of the ankle joints
This is a hinged joint formed between the distal ends of the tibia and fibula and the talus. It only allows *dorsiflexion* and *plantar flexion*. Palpation around the

ankle joints, as well as eliciting signs of inflammation, should also include a careful examination of the *Achilles tendon* for:

1. Nodules (RA, xanthomas, gouty tophi, etc.).
2. Swelling and tenderness (Achilles tendinitis — traumatic or as a manifestation of seronegative arthritis).

Examination of the subtalar (talocalcaneal) joints

This is a complex joint allowing for *inversion* and *eversion* of the foot. Often pain experienced at the ankle emanates from this joint and not the 'true' ankle joint. If pain is elicited on inversion and eversion of the foot (*Fig.* 14.8) it is this joint that is invariably involved. If excessive inversion and/or eversion is elicited at the joint, accompanied by localized tenderness, rupture of one of the many powerful restraining ligaments around this joint should be suspected.

◄ Pain in the ankle is often found to be emanating from the subtalar joint and not the tibiotalar joint ('true' ankle joint).

This joint is frequently affected in rheumatoid arthritis and *valgus* and *varus* deformities are not uncommon and if present lead to an abnormal gait which can result in far-reaching consequences resulting eventually in mechanical damage to the knee and even the hip. Secondary damage in this joint is also seen in rheumatoid arthritis, e.g. a valgus deformity of the knee causing valgus deformity of the ipsilateral subtalar joint is not an uncommon combination.

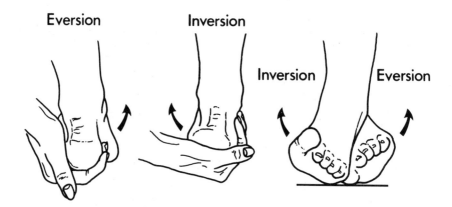

Subtalar joint – range of movement

Fig. 14.8. Testing inversion and eversion of the ankle. This movement occurs at the subtalar joint.

Examination of the mid-tarsal joint(s)
This again is a complex joint allowing rotational and gliding movements. It allows the forefoot to be rotated medially or laterally.

Examination of the tarsometatarsal, the metatarsophalangeal and the interphalangeal joints
Although these are small joints they should always be examined carefully as often significant diagnostic signs will be found within them. Some of these are presented diagrammatically (*Fig.* 14.9).

Examination of the arches of the foot
These are the *medial* (most prominent) and the *lateral*.
These arches are maintained by:
1. Shape of the bony structure
2. Muscles
3. Ligaments
Loss of the medial arch gives rise to flat feet — *pes planus*. Exaggeration of the lateral arch is known as *pes cavus*. The arches are especially important in distributing body weight to the ground and their loss results in abnormal gait and stresses all the structures of the foot causing pain.

◀ Loss of the foot arches results in excessive stress on all the structures of the foot causing pain.

Examination of the thoracic spine
Movement in the thoracic spine is limited and one of its main functions is to provide fixation for the rib cage.

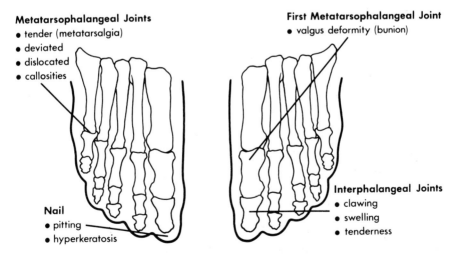

Metatarsophalangeal Joints
- tender (metatarsalgia)
- deviated
- dislocated
- callosities

First Metatarsophalangeal Joint
- valgus deformity (bunion)

Nail
- pitting
- hyperkeratosis

Interphalangeal Joints
- clawing
- swelling
- tenderness

Fig. 14.9.   Joint signs in the foot.

Inspection of the thoracic spine should take particular note of the presence of a *scoliosis* (lateral curvature) or exaggerated *kyphosis* (anterior curvature. An *angulated kyphosis* is known as gibbus and indicates collapse of one or more thoracic vertebrae, and is usually due to old spinal *tuberculous osteomyelitis* (*Pott's disease*), malignant disease or osteoporosis. The presence of a thoracic scoliosis may be secondary to a scoliosis in the lumbar region and in this case the spine describes a gentle letter 'S'. In this case the scoliosis is *compensatory* and will be abolished if the patient is asked to bend forwards. A *fixed thoracic scoliosis* is usually indicative of a congenital abnormality of the spine and/or *paravertebral musculature*. It is also seen in patients who have previously had poliomyelitis affecting the paravertebral muscles.

◄ A compensatory scoliosis is abolished on forward flexion.

One of the more important examinations of the thoracic spine includes measuring *chest expansion*. This should be done with the patient's hands placed comfortably on their head and the tape measure placed around the chest at the fourth intercostal space. The patient is then instructed to breathe in fully. Normal adult expansion should be at least 5–6 cm. It can be severely restricted with *ankylosing spondylitis* but care should be taken in interpretation as chest expansion diminishes with age.

◄ Examination of the thoracic spine should include measurement of chest expansion.

Lumbar spine examination
The lumbar spine is one of the most common sites of symptomatology in rheumatic diseases (*see* Chapter 3) and accurate examination is therefore of the utmost importance.

Inspection should reveal the presence of any abnormal curvatures, e.g. scoliosis, kyphosis or loss or exaggeration of the lumbar lordosis. Loss of the lumbar lordosis is much more significant in a young person than in the older age group, as it progressively flattens out during life.

◄ There is a gradual loss of lumbar lordosis with age.

Palpation of the lumbar spine should include the paravertebral muscles as well as the spinous processes. Particular attention should be paid to any spasm in the paravertebral muscles or localized tenderness over the spinous processes. This is often best elicited by gentle percussion over the spinous processes using the fist of the examining hand.

Movements of the lumbar spine are:
1. Forward flexion ('bend down and touch your toes')

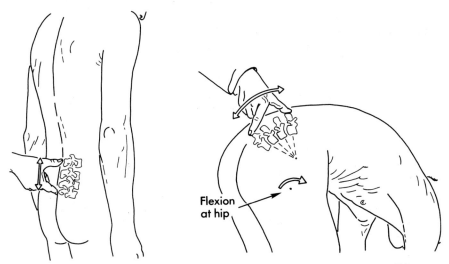

Fig. 14.10. Schober's test to assess lumbar flexion (*see* text for details).

2. Extension ('bend your spine backwards')
3. Lateral flexion ('slide your left/right hand down your left/right thigh')
4. Rotation ('with hands on hips twist round to your right, twist round to your left')

Examination of the movements of the lumbar spine is usually aided by resting a hand gently on the shoulder of the patient during the execution of the various manoeuvres. On forward flexion it is vitally important that flexion of the lumbar spine is being assessed and not flexion at the hip. To do this the thumb is placed on the spinous processes of L1 and the index finger on L4. As the patient flexes forward the thumb and index finger should separate indicating a fanning out of the lumbar spinous processes (*Fig.* 14.10). This is Schober's test (*see* Chapter 7).

The sciatic nerve stretch test (straight leg-raising and Lasegue's sign). Stretching of the sciatic nerve is achieved by raising the extended leg from the couch to 90°. In a normal patient this will be achieved without pain. A patient who has pressure on the sciatic nerve roots, e.g. a prolapsed disc, will attempt to limit the stretching of the sciatic nerve by resisting straight leg-raising. A note should be made of the angle at which resistance is encountered.

Lasegue's sign is a modification of the straight leg-raising test. With the knee flexed at 90°, the hip is flexed to 90° and then the knee slowly extended to the vertical position. Care must be taken in the interpretation of both these tests. Stretching of the hamstring muscles in some patients will produce *localized* pain around the popliteal fossa but pain arising from sciatic nerve radiates down the leg from the buttock.

Sacro-iliac joint examination

Palpation over sacro-iliac joints may reveal localized tenderness and again this is often best achieved by gentle percussion with the fist. The sacro-iliac joints may be stressed by either firm downward pressure over the anterior superior iliac spines with the patient prone, or firm downward pressure over the sacrum with the patient supine. Both these tests result in 'springing' of the pelvis and will be painful if there is inflammation in the sacro-iliac joints or damage to the surrounding ligaments.

Index